Department of Veterans Affairs
Health Services Research & Development Service

Evidence-based Synthesis Program

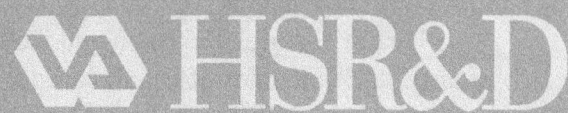

Evidence Synthesis for Determining the Responsiveness of Depression Questionnaires and Optimal Treatment Duration for Antidepressant Medications

I0470821

October 2009

Prepared for:

Department of Veterans Affairs
Veterans Health Administration
Health Services Research
& Development Service
Washington, DC 20420

Prepared by:

Durham Veterans Affairs Medical
Center/Duke Evidence-based
Practice Center
Durham, NC

Investigators:

John W. Williams Jr., MD, MHS
Professor of Medicine and Psychiatry,
Durham VA Medical Center and Duke
University

Director, Evidence-Based Practice Center

Durham, NC

Monica Nora Slubicki, MD
Resident in Psychiatry,
VA Administrative Chief Resident
2009-2010,
Duke University Medical Center

Durham, NC

Damon S. Tweedy, MD
Medical Director, Primary-Care Mental
Health Integration, Durham VA Medical
Center

Consulting Associate, Duke University
Medical Center

Durham, NC

Daniel W. Bradford, MD, MPH
Assistant Professor of Psychiatry,
Durham VA Medical Center and Duke
University Medical Center

Director, Psychosocial Rehabilitation and
Recovery Center, Durham VAMC

Durham, NC

Ranak B. Trivedi, PhD
AHRQ Postdoctoral Fellow in Health
Services Research,
Durham VA Medical Center and Duke
University

Durham, NC

Dana Baker, MS
Clinical Research Coordinator
Duke University

Durham, NC

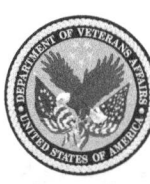

PREFACE

VA's Health Services Research and Development (HSR&D) Service works to improve the cost, quality, and outcomes of health care for our nation's veterans. Collaborating with VA leaders, managers, and policy makers, HSR&D focuses on important healthcare topics that are likely to have significant impact on quality improvement efforts. One significant collaborative effort is HSR&D's Evidence-based Synthesis Program (ESP). Through this program, HSR&D provides timely and accurate evidence syntheses on targeted health care topics. These products will be disseminated broadly throughout VA and will: inform VA clinical policy, develop clinical practice guidelines, set directions for future research to address gaps in knowledge, identify the evidence to support VA performance measures, and rationalize drug formulary decisions.

HSR&D provides funding for four ESP Centers. Each Center has an active and publicly acknowledged VA affiliation and also serves as an Evidence Based Practice Center (EPC) supported by the Agency for Healthcare Research and Quality (AHRQ). The Centers will each generate three evidence syntheses annually on clinical practice topics of key importance to VHA leadership and policymakers. A planning committee with representation from HSR&D, Patient Care Services (PCS), Quality Enhancement Research Initiative (QUERI), Office of Quality and Performance (OQP), and the VISN Clinical and Quality Management Officers, has been established to identify priority topics and key stakeholder concerns and to ensure the quality of final reports. Comments on this evidence report are welcome and can be sent to Susan Schiffner, ESP Program Manager, at Susan.Schiffner@va.gov.

TABLE OF CONTENTS

EXECUTIVE SUMMARY..1

    Background...1

    Methods 1

    Results..2

INTRODUCTION..6

BACKGROUND 7

    Depression Questionnaires 7

    Measuring Responsiveness to Change...7

    Risk of Relapse or Recurrence..8

METHODS 9

    Topic Development..9

    Search Strategy 9

    Study Selection 10

    Data abstraction...11

    Quality Assessment...11

    Data Synthesis...11

    Peer Review..12

RESULTS 12

    Literature Flow..12

    Key Question #1..13

    Key Question #2..17

SUMMARY AND DISCUSSION 20

    Limitations...21

    Conclusions...22

FUTURE RESEARCH...23

TABLES

Table 1..13

Table 2..14

Table 3..14

Table 4..15

Table 5..16

Table 6..18

Table 7..22

FIGURES & APPENDICES

Figure 1..8

Figure 2. 24

Figure 3. 24

Figure 4. 24

Appendix A. Search strategy...25

Appendix B. Full text exclusions...27

Appendix C. Quality ratings..31

Appendix D. Peer review...33

APPENDIX E. Evidence Tables

Evidence Table 1...38

Evidence Table 2...39

Evidence Table 3...40

Evidence Table 4...41

Evidence Table 5...42

REFERENCES...43

EXECUTIVE SUMMARY

BACKGROUND

According to projections from the World Health Organization, depression will be the second leading cause of disability in the developed world by 2020. Primary care clinicians care for approximately two thirds of depressed individuals. In 2000, the U.S. economic burden of depressive disorders was estimated to be 83.1 billion dollars. This included 31% direct medical costs, 7% suicide-related mortality costs, and 62% workplace costs. A variety of strategies have been tested to improve patient outcomes. Among these, integrated care models have emerged as both effective and cost effective. A recent systematic review identifies symptom monitoring as a key element of these integrated care models. However, the review did not identify the standardized depression scales that are responsive to clinically important change.

A separate but important issue raised by Veterans Administration (VA) Stakeholders is how long to continue antidepressant medication for patients who respond to acute phase treatment. Clinical guidelines recommend continuation treatment for 4-6 months for uncomplicated major depression and some national performance measures are linked to these guidelines. However, clinical guidelines for longer-term maintenance phase treatment are more variable and performance indicators (e.g., Healthcare Effectiveness Data and Information Set, HEDIS) do not address maintenance phase treatment. A better understanding of the evidence for long-term treatment efficacy with antidepressants would inform guidelines and performance measurement.

The Key Questions (KQ) were:

KQ1: In patients with major depressive disorder treated in primary care settings, what assessment tools are responsive to change? This review should specifically address instruments that are feasible for the primary care setting.

KQ2: In primary care patients with major depressive disorder who remit with antidepressant medication, what is the minimum treatment duration to decrease the risk of relapse or recurrence? This review will focus on patients without comorbid substance abuse, PTSD, psychosis or other conditions where guidelines would recommend specialty based care.

METHODS

We searched PubMed from 1950-2009 using standard search terms; PsychInfo was also searched for key question one (KQ1). Additional citations were identified from reference lists. Titles, abstracts, and articles were reviewed in duplicate by physicians trained in the critical analysis of literature. For KQ1, we included primary literature comparing one of the 6 eligible depression symptom questionnaires to an interview-based reference standard. For key question two (KQ2), we searched for and identified a high quality systematic review, then searched for relevant randomized trials published since the original review (2007-2009). For eligible articles, data were extracted in duplicate. We evaluated study quality for the primary literature and the systematic review. All data were summarized narratively. An overall strength of evidence "GRADE" was assigned to the body of evidence for each key question.

RESULTS

For KQ1, we screened 743 titles, rejected 661, and performed a more detailed review on 82 articles. From these, we identified 3 unduplicated observational studies meeting eligibility criteria. For KQ2, we screened 154 titles, rejected 139, and performed a more detailed review on 15 articles. From these, we identified 1 recent high quality systematic review and 3 relevant randomized controlled trials (RCTs).

KEY QUESTION 1. In patients with major depressive disorder treated in primary care settings, what assessment tools are responsive to change?

We identified 3 studies evaluating the responsiveness of the Patient Heath Questionnaire-9 (PHQ-9), in primary care patients with depressive disorders; no studies for the other eligible questionnaires were identified. A total of 2,330 patients were evaluated, one study was limited to older adults and one included VA settings.

The most relevant study to VA settings and patients was a high quality secondary analysis from the IMPACT study, a randomized trial comparing collaborative care to usual care. In this study, participants were ≥ 60 years old, had a mean of 3.8 chronic diseases and a research-based diagnosis of major depression or dysthymia. Three of the eighteen primary care sites were VA. The analysis was limited to the 434 patients in the intervention arm with complete assessments at baseline, 3- and 6-month follow-up. Responsiveness was reported as the standardized response mean (SRM) which is calculated as: Mean (time 2) - Mean (time1)/standard deviation of score changes.

For the cohort overall, the mean change and standardized response mean at 3 months was: -7.5±5.8, SRM -1.3 (95% CI -1.4 to -1.2). At 6 months, the mean change and SRM were: -8.0±6.1, SRM -1.3 (95% CI –1.4 to -1.2). Responsiveness equaled or exceeded the longer Symptom Checklist-20 (SCL-20, self-administered 20-item questionnaire measuring depressive symptoms) at these two time points. Results were not significantly different when restricted to patients with major depressive disorder (MDD). For the 317 patients with MDD, an independent, structured diagnostic assessment was used to classify patients at six month follow-up as: persistent MDD, partial- or full remission. Greater clinical improvement was associated with larger reductions in PHQ-9 scores. The mean change and SRM for each group was: persistent MDD -5.6±6.6, SRM -0.8; partial remission -8.4±6.1, SRM -1.4; full remission -9.8±5.9, SRM -1.7. In this analysis, the SRM was again similar for the PHQ-9 and SCL-20. An analysis to determine the minimum clinically important difference (MCID), estimated this value conservatively at 4.78, meaning a 5-point or larger decline in the PHQ-9 indicates clinically meaningful improvement.

Two fair quality studies, conducted with a German language version of the PHQ-9 showed similar results at 3- and 12-month follow-ups. Standardized response means ranged from -1.42 to -2.15 for patients rated as responders by a structured interview. One study conducted subgroup analyses and found similar responsiveness for men and women, different age groups, depression diagnosis and presence or absence of comorbid physical illness.

2

These three studies differed in a variety of design features that could lead to heterogeneous results including: study quality, questionnaire language, follow-up timing, and participant characteristics. Despite these sources of potential variability, the overall results were consistent across studies. The PHQ-9 is responsive to clinically important changes in symptom status. Using the GRADE criteria, we judged the overall quality of evidence for this finding as moderate. For the finding that the minimum clinically important difference is 5, the quality of evidence is low based on a single, albeit, high quality studies.

A recent literature synthesis identified longitudinal assessment of depression symptoms with a standardized scale as a critical component of effective depression care. The PHQ-9 is the best validated scale in primary care populations, both for initial diagnosis and for detecting response to change. Its routine use for measuring response to treatment could improve patient care and outcomes, but logistical support to integrate the questionnaire into clinical practice would likely be needed to achieve successful implementation.

- The PHQ-9 is the best validated instrument for detecting clinically important response to treatment. Quality of Evidence = Moderate
- A 5 point change on the PHQ-9 is estimated as the minimum clinically important difference. Quality of Evidence = Low

KEY QUESTION 2. In primary care patients with major depressive disorder who remit with antidepressant medication, what is the minimum treatment duration to decrease the risk of relapse or recurrence?

We included 1 applicable high quality systematic review and 3 RCT's with 4 comparisons published since the systematic review. A total of 9,024 patients in 26 RCT's were evaluated. None of the studies included a VA setting; three were restricted to patients age ≥ 65 years old.

The systematic review evaluated 23 fair quality RCT's comparing second-generation antidepressant to placebo in fully- or partially-remitted patients. Patients with comorbid psychiatric or serious medical conditions were generally excluded. Twelve took place in unspecified outpatient clinics, four in primary care and psychiatry clinics, and the remaining seven did not specify the setting. Relapse or recurrence was generally defined using a predefined score on the Hamilton Depression Rate Scale (HDRS), a validated, interview-administered depression severity measure. The authors stratified the studies according to treatment duration: less than 1 year after acute phase treatment remission (continuation) and 1 year or more after acute phase treatment duration (maintenance). The unadjusted frequency of relapse for continuation phase (12 studies) was 22% for active treatment and 42% for placebo. In a pooled analysis the relative risk of relapse was 0.54 (95% CI 0.46 to 0.62); heterogeneity was moderate ($I2 =47\%$). The unadjusted frequency of recurrence for maintenance phase (11 studies) was similar to shorter duration studies, 26% with active treatment and 48% with placebo. The relative risk of recurrence was 0.56 (95% CI 0.48 to 0.66); heterogeneity was moderate ($I2 =30\%$). Loss to follow up due to adverse events was not significantly different between antidepressant and placebo. Only one study out of the 23 RCT's randomized patients in remission to varying durations (14, 38 or 50 weeks) of continuation phase antidepressant or placebo. In that study, relapse rates were significantly lower for patients on active treatment at 14 weeks (26% vs. 49%), and 38 weeks (9% vs. 23%) but not at 50 weeks (11% vs. 16%). In meta-regression analyses, the duration of treatment prior to and after randomization were not associated with the magnitude of treatment effect, suggesting a constant reduction in relative risk.

Of the three additional RCT's identified, the PREVENT study was the most informative. This multi-phase, double-blind, placebo-controlled study evaluated 12 and 24 month treatment with venlafaxine ER versus placebo. It found that venlafaxine ER was associated with a statistically significantly lower recurrence rate at 12-month follow-up (23.1% vs. 42.0%). Using an expanded definition of recurrence, freedom from recurrence at 24 month follow up was 67% for venlafaxine vs. 41.0% for placebo. The 24 month PREVENT follow up phase did not report on patients lost to follow up. Another good quality RCT reported the results of a 24 week RCT of escitalopram (10-20mg/day) versus placebo in older adults who had responded to acute treatment with escitalopram for MDD. Escitalopram was associated with a significantly lower relapse rate compared with placebo (9% vs. 33%, p<0.001). The last RCT evaluated was a small, fair quality trial that did not find a significant difference between antidepressant and placebo for prevention of relapse.

The high quality systematic review and 2 of the most recent relevant RCT's provide moderately strong evidence that continued antidepressant treatment decreases the risk of subsequent relapse for patients with MDD who achieve partial- or full-remission. The moderate strength of evidence grade is based on RCT's with some important methodological limitations, generally consistent results, and a precise estimate of effect. Of note, none of these studies were performed in a VA population. The magnitude of risk reduction was similar for shorter- and longer-term trials and maintained for up to 2.5 years. However, these trials do not directly address the question about the minimum duration of continued antidepressant treatment since they report the average risk reduction over these time periods. At the individual patient level, the decision for how long to continue antidepressant treatment should be based on effectiveness, adverse effects and patient preferences. Additional studies that could include decision analyses and randomized trials that stratify treatment duration based on risk factors are needed to inform clinical guidelines and performance measures for maintenance phase treatment.

- A high quality systematic review and 2 of the most recent relevant RCT's provide moderately strong evidence that continued antidepressant treatment decreases the risk of subsequent relapse for patients with MDD who achieve partial- or full-remission. Continued treatment for 1 to 2 years after achieving partial- or full-remission with second-generation antidepressants decreases the risk of relapse or recurrence by almost 50%. The number needed to treat to prevent one relapse was 5. Quality of Evidence = Moderate.

- The magnitude of risk reduction was similar for shorter- and longer-term trials and maintained for up to 2 years. However, these trials do not directly address the minimum duration of continued antidepressant treatment since they report the average risk reduction over these time periods.

Determining the Responsiveness of Depression Questionnaires and
Optimal Treatment Duration for Antidepressant Medications

Evidence-based Synthesis Program

EVIDENCE REPORT

INTRODUCTION

According to projections from the World Health Organization, depression will be the second leading cause of disability in the developed world by 2020.[1] Primary care clinicians (PCCs) care for approximately two thirds of depressed individuals.[2] Rates of guideline concordant care for depression, however, are suboptimal and patient outcomes are often poor.[3, 4] A variety of strategies have been tested to improve patient outcomes including: physician education, continuous quality improvement, and reorganizing care to integrate mental health and primary care. Of these approaches, integrated care models have been found to be both effective and cost effective.[5-7] A recent analysis using meta-regression techniques identified baseline and follow-up assessments of depressive symptoms with a standardized scale as critical components of successful integrated models.[8] Patients randomized to integrated care are more likely to receive an adequate trial of antidepressants and/or empirically based psychotherapies and are approximately twice as likely to respond to treatment compared to usual care. Much like serial monitoring of Hemoglobin A1c in patients with diabetes, careful symptom assessment through standardized depression scales may facilitate treatment changes that improve outcomes. However, the review did not identify the standardized scales that are responsive to clinically important change.

A second issue relevant to the primary care management of depression is the optimal duration of antidepressant medication. For patients who remit with treatment, the benefits of sustained antidepressant medication to prevent relapse or recurrence must be balanced against the risks. Early clinical guidelines recommended 4-6 months of continuation phase treatment for uncomplicated major depression due to high rates of early relapse and demonstrated efficacy of continuation treatment. Maintenance phase treatment is recommended for patients at high risk for recurrence. More recently, some guidelines[9, 10] have recommended longer duration of continuation phase treatment despite emerging evidence about potential long-term adverse effects including gastrointestinal bleeding [11] and osteoporosis.[12, 13] The duration of antidepressant medication treatment not only has important implications for individual patients, but also has cost implications that include the direct cost of medication, longitudinal monitoring and treatment of adverse effects.

To inform recommendations for clinical guidelines and potential performance measures, this evidence synthesis evaluates the responsiveness of depression questionnaires feasible for primary care settings and data from randomized trials that examine the effects on continued antidepressant use to prevent relapse or recurrence.

BACKGROUND

DEPRESSION QUESTIONNAIRES

A prior systematic review identified eleven self-administered depression questionnaires that had been evaluated in primary care settings; most have been evaluated in VA settings.[14] Questionnaires ranged from 1 to 30 items; 7 had versions of ≤ 10 items. Response formats included "yes/no," frequency ratings, and statements of symptom severity. Scores ranged from as brief as 0 to 1 for a single item, "yes/no" questionnaire to 0-100. All instruments could be self-administered in < 5 minutes but interview administration varied more substantially due to differences in length and response format. Six of the instruments were considered useful for monitoring severity or response but this judgment was based on scale characteristics rather than empirical data. A recent update of identified 3 additional questionnaires and new studies for existing questionnaires.[15] Brief, 2-9-item questionnaires compared comparably to longer questionnaires.[16] The review concluded that the Patient Health Questionnaire-9 (PHQ-9) had better performance characteristics and gave more information for depression diagnosis than other instruments. A recent National Heart, Lung, and Blood Institute working group recommended the PHQ-2 (whose items are contained within the PHQ-9) to screen for trial entry and recommended the interviewer-rated Hamilton Depression Rating Scale (HDRS) to assess outcomes. Interviewer-rated instruments, such as the Hamilton, are the reference standard for evaluating depression severity but require greater expertise, training and administration time than self-administered questionnaires and for this reason are not considered feasible for clinical purposes in the primary care setting.[17] Given the large number of validated questionnaires, we focused this review on brief instruments that may be more acceptable to clinicians and patients.

Brief Depression Questionnaires Validated in Primary Care Settings

Questionnaire	Items	Response format	Literacy level
BDI Fast Screen	7	4 Statements of symptom severity	Easy
CES-D	10	4 Frequency ratings: "less than 1d" to "most or all (5-7d)"	Easy
DEPS	10	4 Frequency ratings: "not at all" to "extremely)"	Average
GDS	15	Yes or no	Easy
PHQ-9	9	4 Frequency ratings: "not at all" to "nearly every day"	Average
SDDS-PC	5	Yes or no	Easy

Abbreviations: BDI, Beck Depression Inventory; CES-D, Center for epidemiologic Studies Depression Screen; DEPS, Depression Scale; GDS, Geriatric Depression Scale; PHQ-9, Patient Health Questionnaire-9; SDDS-PC, Symptom-Driven Diagnostic System for Primary Care

MEASURING RESPONSIVENESS TO CHANGE

Health status measures are typically evaluated for reliability and validity. A third characteristic, important for detecting clinically important change over time, is the measure's responsiveness.

Responsiveness is determined by two properties: reproducibility, and the ability to register changes in scores when a patient's symptom status shows clinically important improvement or deterioration. Although there is no universally recommended measure of responsiveness, most indices rely on calculation of an effect size. The effect size is a unit-free index that uses the mean change score in the numerator and a measure of variability in the denominator. The Standardized Response Mean[18] and the Responsiveness Index[19, 20] are particularly useful approaches to calculating effect sizes for this application because they incorporate information about the response variance into the denominator. Deyo and others argue that the issue is not just sensitivity to change but the ability to discriminate between those who improve and those who do not.[19, 21] Receiver operating characteristic curves are proposed as an approach for describing how well various changes in scale scores can distinguish between improved and unimproved patients. This approach requires a valid reference standard to make these clinical classifications.

RISK OF RELAPSE OR RECURRENCE

The goal of depression treatment is to help patients achieve full recovery, defined as a sustained period where no or minimal symptoms exist and full functional status has returned. Operationally, this has been defined as a Hamilton Depression Rating Scale score of ≤ 7. [22] Patients with major depression who remit with antidepressant medication have at least a 50% lifetime risk of recurrence. Patients at particularly high risk include those with ≥ 2 prior major depressive episodes, chronic major depression, a family history of bipolar disorder and more severe depression. The 1993 Agency for Health Care Policy and Research clinical guideline for depression used epidemiological data to propose three treatment phases: acute, continuation and maintenance (Figure).[23] Acute phase treatment describes the period of initial treatment until remission is achieved, continuation phase extends treatment for 4 to 6 months to prevent early relapse, and maintenance phase treatment continues for 1 or more years for selected patients at increased of recurrence.

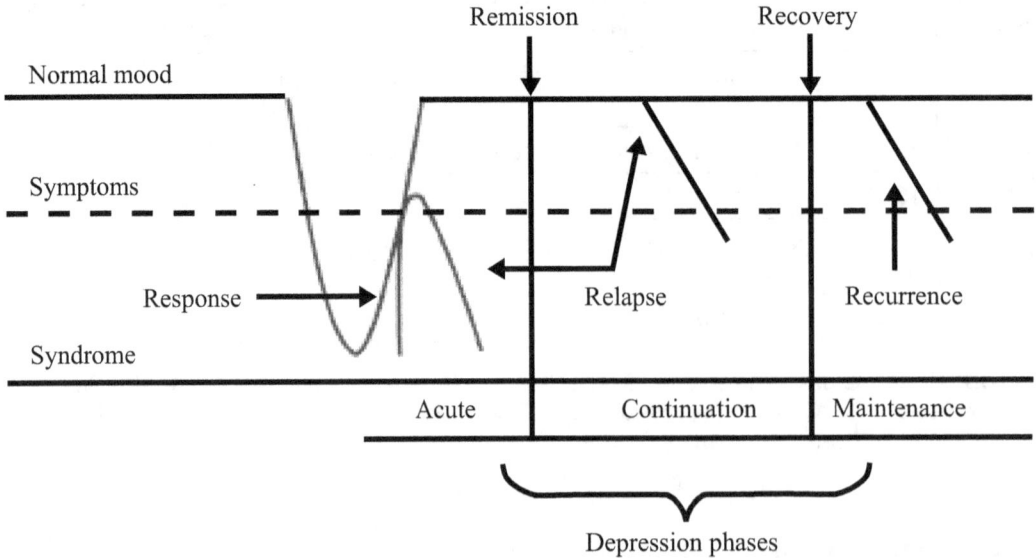

Figure 1. Phases of Depression Treatment

Current guidelines provide a range of recommendations for continuation and maintenance phase treatment. For example, the National Institute for Clinical Excellence guidelines (developed by the British National Health Service) recommend ≥ 2 years treatment for patients with 2 or more major depressive episodes accompanied by functional impairment, while the Institute for Clinical Systems Improvement guidelines, a US regional health care collaborative, recommend 6 -12 months treatment without specifying which groups should get longer duration of treatment.[9, 10] Since these guidelines were published, new data from randomized trials provide additional evidence on the benefits of antidepressant medication for preventing relapse or recurrence. In addition, systematic reviews provide evidence on potential long-term risks of continuing antidepressant medication.

METHODS

TOPIC DEVELOPMENT

The Veterans Health Administration (VA) uses quality improvement strategies including clinical practice guidelines, clinical reminders in the electronic medical record and performance measurement to improve care processes. For veterans with depression and other mental illnesses managed in primary care settings, the VA has recently made major investments in integrated primary care-mental health programs. This project was nominated by Ira Katz, Deputy Chief, Patient Care Services for Mental Health and Carla Cassidy and Joe Francis, Office of Quality and Performance with input from a technical expert panel, and assigned to the Durham VA Evidence Synthesis Team. The overall goal was to synthesize data on two key issues – the responsiveness of depression severity instruments and minimum duration of treatment with antidepressants – to inform future quality improvement efforts.

The final key questions (KQ) are:

KQ1: In patients with major depressive disorder treated in primary care settings, what assessment tools are responsive to change? This review should specifically address instruments that are feasible for the primary care setting.

KQ2: In primary care patients with major depressive disorder who remit with antidepressant medication, what is the minimum treatment duration to decrease the risk of relapse or recurrence? This review will focus on patients without comorbid substance abuse, post-traumatic stress disorder, psychosis or other conditions where guidelines would recommend specialty based care.

SEARCH STRATEGY

We conducted a search in Medline and PsychInfo for literature published from 1950 through February 2009. For key question one (KQ1), we searched for relevant primary literature. For key question two (KQ2), our search strategy was designed to identify recent high quality systematic reviews and any relevant randomized controlled trials published since the review. A high quality review was identified that included articles published through March 2007; our search for additional randomized controlled trials (RCT) included articles published from January 2007 through February 2009. Appendix A provides the search strategy in detail. We reviewed reference lists of pertinent studies for additional citations. All citations were imported into an electronic database (EndNote X1).

STUDY SELECTION

Two trained researchers reviewed the titles and/or abstracts of citations identified from literature searches. Full-text articles of potentially relevant citations were retrieved for further review. Each article was reviewed with a brief screening form (see Appendix B) to determine eligibility and record reasons for exclusion. In case of disagreement, the two reviewers met to identify and resolve the disagreement. Eligible articles had English-language abstracts and provided primary data relevant to the key questions. Eligibility criteria varied depending on the question of interest, as described below.

To be included in our evidence report for KQ1, a study had to:
- Evaluate Beck Depression Fast Screen [24], Center for Epidemiologic Studies Depression Scale 10-item version [25], DEPS scale [26,]Geriatric Depression Scale 15 item version [27], the Patient Heath Questionnaire-9[28], or Symptom Driven Diagnostic System-PC [29]
- Compare the depression questionnaire to an interview-based depression severity assessment such as the Hamilton Depression Rating Scale or Clinical Global Impression
- Use a longitudinal study design so that response to change could be assessed
- Be conducted in adult patients with depressive disorder followed in the outpatient setting and
- Be published in English

We restricted the depression questionnaires to those that had been identified in a previous systematic review[14, 15] as having adequate performance characteristics to identify patients with major depression in primary care settings, had a range of scores sufficient to show change and that were feasible for use as self- or interviewer administered instruments. Thus, questionnaires with a very limited scoring range (e.g. Yale, PRIME-MD) or with greater than 10 items (e.g., 21 item Beck Depression Inventory, 21 item Center for Epidemiologic Depression Scale, Hopkins Symptom Checklist) were not considered. Although the Geriatric Depression Scale is 15 items, we included this measure because it is specifically cited as an option in the VA/DOD Major Depression Guideline.

To be included in our evidence report for KQ2, a study had to:
- Be a systematic review of randomized controlled trials. A review was considered systematic if it contained a methods section describing the search strategy and described an analytic approach to data synthesis.
- Focus on adult patients with major depressive disorder who remitted or improved substantially with antidepressant medication.
- Compared continuation or maintenance phase treatment with antidepressant medication to placebo.
- Report relapse and/or recurrence rates.
- Be published in English.

We then applied quality criteria (see below) and retained the most recent high quality systematic review. We included newly identified studies if they were randomized controlled trials, instead of reviews, and if they met all other criteria described for systematic reviews

DATA ABSTRACTION

We abstracted the following data from included studies: Study Design/setting, eligibility criteria/method for assembling cohort, exclusion criteria, sample size, duration of follow-up, demographics, clinical category/baseline depression, results and conclusions. For KQ 1, we also abstracted information on the method of administration and version of depression questionnaire and on the interview-based depression evaluation. For KQ2, we also abstracted information on the intervention and comparator and follow-up rate. Data abstractions were completed by a single reviewer, then over-read for accuracy by 1-2 additional reviewers. Any disagreements were resolved by discussion and consensus.

QUALITY ASSESSMENT

To assess internal validity of studies, we used criteria appropriate to the study design (see Appendix C). For KQ1, we abstracted data on whether the interview-based assessment was performed blind to the depression questionnaire results; whether the depression questionnaire was performed blind to the interview-based assessment; whether the interview-based assessment was adequate; the completeness of follow-up; whether the analytic methods were appropriate; study funding; and whether a conflict of interest statement was given.

For KQ2, we abstracted data for systematic reviews and separately for randomized controlled trials. For systematic reviews, we abstracted search methods and strategy; whether inclusion/ exclusion criteria were clearly defined and appropriate; whether primary studies were appropriately evaluated for quality; were the assessments reproducible; was there an analysis of variability; were results combined appropriately; was publication bias assessed; were clinically important outcomes, including harms and benefits, reported. For randomized trials, we determined whether the method of randomization and allocation concealment was adequate; whether intervention and control groups were similar at baseline regarding the most important prognostic indicators; was the outcome assessed using a valid methodology and the assessor blinded; was the care provider blinded; was the patient blinded; was loss to follow-up < 20% and differential loss between groups < 10%; were missing outcome data addressed adequately; and was there a conflict of interest.

DATA SYNTHESIS

We constructed evidence tables showing the study characteristics and results for all included studies, organized by key question. We critically analyzed studies to compare their characteristics, methods, and findings. We compiled a summary of findings for each key question or clinical topic, and drew conclusions based on qualitative synthesis of the findings. We assigned an overall quality of evidence using the GRADE criteria.[30]

PEER REVIEW

A draft version of this report was sent to four peer reviewers. Their comments and our responses
are presented in Appendix D.

RESULTS

LITERATURE FLOW

For KQ1, the combined library contained 673 citations, of which we reviewed 82 articles at the
full-text level (Figure 2.). Of the 82 articles, 4 studies met eligibility criteria [31-34] but two
citations [31, 32] were derived from the same study population leaving 3 unique studies. For
KQ2, the combined library for systematic reviews contained 106 citations, of which we reviewed
9 articles at the full-text level (Figure 3). Of the 9 articles, we included the most recent, high
quality review meeting eligibility criteria. [35] To identify new studies since the eligible
systematic review was complete, we searched for relevant RCT's from January 2007 to present.
This search identified 48 citations, of which we reviewed 6 articles at the full-text level (Figure
4.). Of the 6 articles, 3 studies with 4 comparisons met eligibility criteria.[36-39]

KEY QUESTION 1

STUDIES EVALUATING RESPONSIVENESS OF DEPRESSION QUESTIONNAIRES

We identified 3 studies that compared change scores for an eligible depression questionnaire to an interview based assessment of depression severity. All three studies used the PHQ-9 and one of these completed a separate analysis of the PHQ-2. Two studies were conducted in Germany, using German language versions of the questionnaire. One study was a secondary analysis from a multi-center randomized trial of care management in older adults and included three VA sites. Key features of the studies are summarized in the Table below and study details are contained in Appendix E.

Table 1: Characteristics of Studies Evaluating Responsiveness of the PHQ-9

Study	Lowe 2004[34]	Lowe 2006[33]	Lowe 2004[32] and Lowe 2005[31]
N	434	1788	108
Primary care	Yes	Mixed	Mixed
VA settings	Yes	No	No
Mean age (SD)	70.9 (7.3)	50.3 (14.7)	41.1 (14.2) to 42.8 (12.1)
Men	160 (36%)	594 (33.2%)	34 (31.5%)
Major depressive disorder	317 (73%)	757 (42.3%)	55 (51%)
Questionnaire	PHQ-9 (English)	PHQ-9 (German)	PHQ-9 (German)
Comparator	Structured Clinical Interview for DSM-IV	Clinical Global Impression	Structured Clinical Interview for DSM-IV
Quality	Good	Fair	Fair

The responsiveness, or sensitivity to change of an instrument describes its ability to accurately detect clinically meaningful change when it occurs. There is no consensus on the best measure for describing responsiveness but three common methods are used in the studies reviewed: effect size, standardized response mean and responsiveness index.

- Effect size: Mean (time 2)-Mean (time1)/Standard deviation (time 1) [40]
- Standardized response mean: Mean (time 2)-Mean (time1)/Standard deviation of score changes [18]
- Responsiveness index: Mean (time 2)-Mean (time1)/Standard deviation in unchanged subjects [19, 20]

The good quality study by Lowe et al [34] is the most applicable to Veterans. It evaluated the responsiveness of the PHQ-9 and Symptom Checklist-20 (SCL) in older adults enrolled in a randomized trial comparing collaborative care to usual care. The PHQ-9 was self-administered or given by telephone interview. The study was conducted in 18 primary care sites, three that were VA. Participants were age ≥ 60 years old, had a mean of 3.8 ± 2.0 chronic diseases and had a research-based diagnosis of major depressive disorder or dysthymia. Among intervention patients, 71% had ≥ 2 prior episodes of depression, 35% screened positive for cognitive impairment and 28% screened positive for anxiety symptoms. Important exclusion criteria were: severe cognitive impairment, CAGE ≥ 2 or history of bipolar disorder or psychosis. The analysis was limited to patients in the intervention arm who had the depression questionnaires, the interview-based Structured Clinical Interview for DSM-IV and clinical assessment within 2 weeks of each other at each scheduled assessment: baseline, 3- and 6-month follow-up. Of the 906 intervention patients, 434 (47.9%) had complete assessments. Study strengths were: independent, blind comparison of the questionnaires and interview-based assessments, an adequate criterion standard and appropriate analysis. A weakness was that only 48% of patients enrolled were analyzed, but the study sample was similar to the intervention group overall except for a smaller proportion of ethnic minorities. The mean change and standardized response mean (SRM) for the PHQ-9 and SLC-20 are shown below:

Table 2. Responsiveness in Patients with Major Depressive Disorder or Dysthymia (n=434)

	Baseline	3 Month Change		6 Month Change	
Instrument	Mean (SD)	Mean (SD)	SRM (95% CI)	Mean (SD)	SRM (95% CI)
PHQ-9, range 0-27	13.6 (5.4)	-7.5 (5.8)	-1.3 (-1.4 to -1.2)	-8.0 (6.1)	-1.3 (-1.4 to -1.2)
SCL-20, range 0-4	1.7 (0.6)	-0.6 (0.7)	-0.9 (-1.0 to -0.8)	-0.8 (0.7)	-1.2 (-1.4 to -1.1)

At 3 months, the PHQ-9 was more responsive than the longer SCL-20; at 6-months the responsiveness was not significantly different. The results were unchanged when the analysis was restricted to subjects with MDD. In a secondary analysis, the SCID was used to categorize treatment response for the 317 patients with MDD as persistent MDD (≥ 5 criterion symptoms), partial remission (1-4 criterion symptoms) or full remission (no criterion symptoms). Using this classification, the mean change and standardized response mean at six months were as follows:

Table 3. Responsiveness Characteristics in Patients with Major Depressive Disorder at Six Month Follow-up (n=317)

	PHQ-9		SCL-20	
SCID category	Mean change (SD)	Standardized response mean	Mean change (SD)	Standardized response mean
Persistent MDD	-5.6 (6.6)	-0.8	-0.3 (0.7)	-0.4
Partial remission	-8.4 (6.1)	-1.4	-0.9 (0.6)	-1.5
Full remission	-9.8 (5.9)	-1.7	-1.3 (0.6)	-2.2

For both instruments, an independent assessment of clinical improvement is associated with greater reductions in symptom scores. Finally, the authors determined the minimum clinically important difference (MCID) in a subset of 82 patients who had the PHQ-9 administered twice, exactly 7 days apart at the 6-month follow-up. The MCID was calculated as the standard error of measurement * 1.96. A sensitivity analysis showed the MCID ranged from 2.59 to 4.78 consistent with prior recommendations based on cross-sectional studies.[41]

The studies by Lowe et al conducted in Germany and using a German-language version of the PHQ-9 are less applicable to VA settings. [31-33] German language versions of the PHQ-9 may theoretically perform differently from the English language version. The larger study [33] enrolled 1878 patients and was conducted in the context of an open-label, post-marketing surveillance trial of sertraline. Patients were adults with major, minor or other depressive disorders beginning a course of the antidepressant sertraline. The PHQ-9 was compared to the Clinical Global Impression (CGI) at 3 months. Patients with a CGI of 1 (very much improved) or 2 (much improved) were classified as responders (n=1552, 86.8%). Study strengths were: a follow-up rate of 95%, and appropriate analysis and administration of the PHQ-9 blind to the CGI results. Study weaknesses were: the CGI criterion standard was applied with knowledge of the PHQ-9 results and almost 50% the raters were non-mental health professionals with a single training session on using the CGI rating scale. In addition the study team included a biostatistician from Pfizer and Pfizer funded the analysis by Lowe et al and the PHQ-9 development suggesting a potential conflict of interest. The mean change scores and standardized response means are shown for CGI responders and non-responders.

Table 4. Responsiveness Characteristics at Three Month Follow-up (n=1788)

CGI category	PHQ-9 (German Language Version)	
	Mean change (95% CI)	Standardized response mean
Non-responder	-4.42 (-5.0 to -3.84)	-1.00
Responder	-11.15 (-11.41 to -10.8)	-2.15

Subgroup analyses were conducted comparing responsiveness by gender, age groups, depression diagnosis, and presence of comorbid physical illness. Standardized response means were similar for these subgroups. Because this study was an open label trial, the study population may be more representative of typical patients initiating antidepressants than those recruited into a randomized trial.

The second German-language evaluation of the PHQ-9 followed a cohort of 167 patients with major depressive disorder (n=55), other depressive disorder (n=53) or no depressive disorder (n=59).[31, 32] Only the first two groups with depressive disorders are relevant to our study question and our discussion is limited to these groups. At 12-months, PHQ-9 changes scores were compared to clinical status as determined by the Structured Clinical Interview for DSM-IV (SCID). Improved status included patients who transitioned from major depressive disorder to other- or no depressive disorder and patients with other depressive disorder who transitioned to no depressive disorder. Worse clinical status included those who transitioned from no depressive disorder to major depressive disorder. Study strengths include a follow-up rate > 80%, appropriate analysis and an adequate criterion standard administered by trained raters with excellent inter-rater reliability. Limitations are lack of an independent, blind comparison between the PHQ-9 and SCID at 12-month follow-up. Results are given for both the PHQ-9 and for its first 2 items (PHQ-2).

Table 5. Responsiveness Characteristics at Twelve Month Follow-up (n=108)

SCID category	PHQ-9			PHQ-2		
	Mean change (SD)	Effect size	Standardized response mean	Mean change (SD)	Effect size	Standardized response mean
Worse	3.25 (4.3)	0.62	0.75	1.0 (2.0)	0.6	0.5
Unchanged MDD Other Depression	0.24 (4.2) -1.96 (5.28)	0.05 -0.38	0.06 -0.37	0.4 (1.3) -0.7 (2.2)	0.3 -0.5	0.3 -0.3
Improved	-6.7 (4.91)	-1.33	-1.42	-2.3 (2.1)	-1.4	-1.1

Across the three studies, the standardized response mean ranged from -1.0 to 0.5 for patients who were unchanged or worse, and -2.15 to -1.4 for those who responded or remitted. Mean changes in PHQ-9 showed greater variability: -5.6 to 3.25 for non-responders and -11.15 to -6.7 for those who responded or remitted. The three studies vary on a number important design factors that may explain some of the observed heterogeneity. Effect sizes were calculated over a range of follow-up from 3 to 12 months. Study samples differed in ways that could affect responsiveness, including the proportion with major depressive disorder, the mean age and proportion male. The PHQ-9 was administered in English and German languages. The interview-based comparator differed and definitions of response varied across studies. Finally, study quality differed importantly. Despite these sources of potential variability, the overall results were consistent across studies. Greater clinical improvement as determined by an interview based severity measure was associated with greater improvement on the PHQ-9. Using the GRADE criteria that incorporates study design, consistency and precision of results, publication bias and directness, we judge the body of evidence as moderate quality, downgrading for limitations in study design.

KEY QUESTION 2

The selected systematic review[35] evaluated 23 fair quality RCT's that compared a second-generation antidepressant to placebo in patients who achieved partial- or full remission after acute phase treatment. Using the quality assessment instrument described in Appendix D, this systematic review met all quality criteria. Included studies generally enrolled patients with a criteria-based diagnosis of major depressive disorder and excluded patients with concurrent psychiatric illness (e.g. substance abuse or anxiety disorder) or severe chronic medical conditions. None of the studies described a VA recruitment site. Four studies recruited patients from primary care and psychiatry outpatient clinics, 12 were conducted in unspecified outpatient clinics; the remaining seven settings were not described. Studies used a randomized discontinuation design, randomizing responders to continued antidepressant or placebo. In all trials, antidepressants were used in the acute phase of treatment; none described adjunctive treatment with non-pharmacological treatment. All but two[42, 43] of the 23 RCT's continued the same antidepressant or antidepressants at the same dose from acute phase treatment to continuation and maintenance phases. Only studies evaluating second-generation antidepressants were included; a list of these is available in the evidence table (Appendix E). The primary outcomes were relapse and recurrence rates during continuation and maintenance phases. Relapse was generally defined as a Hamilton Depression Rating Scale score exceeding a specified severity level. Secondary outcomes were adverse event rates and treatment discontinuation due to adverse events. A separate analysis included 4 RCT's that compared antidepressants to each other with regards to rates of relapse after remission; this analysis is not included for further discussion here because it does not relate directly to KQ2.

Because the RCT's defined their continuation and maintenance phases differently, the authors of the systematic review stratified the studies by treatment duration: less than 1 year after acute phase treatment remission (continuation) and 1 year or more after acute phase treatment remission (maintenance). Results stratified by continuation and maintenance phase treatment are summarized in Table 6. The unadjusted frequency of relapse for continuation phase (12 studies) was 22% for active treatment and 42% for placebo. Heterogeneity among these trials was moderate ($I^2 = 47\%$). The unadjusted frequency of recurrence for maintenance phase (11 studies) was similar to continuation phase treatment: 26% for active treatment and 48% placebo. Heterogeneity for these longer duration studies was also moderate ($I^2 = 30\%$). Tests for publication bias were not statistically significant for either group of studies. Meta-regression analyses were conducted to evaluate heterogeneity. The duration of open-label treatment before random assignment of responders, the length of the post-randomization phase and type of second-generation antidepressant were not associated with the estimate of effect. The authors concluded that their results provide consistent evidence in favor of antidepressant treatment over placebo in both continuation and maintenance phases.

Table 6. Systematic Review -Summary of findings

	Unadjusted frequency of relapse/recurrence	Pooled relative risk of relapse/ recurrence	Number needed to treat to prevent 1 additional relapse/ recurrence
Continuation (<1yr of ongoing treatment)	22% antidepressant 42% placebo	0.54 (95% CI 0.46 to 0.62)	5 (95% CI 4 to 6) over a mean time of 8 months
Maintenance (≥1yr ongoing treatment)	26% antidepressant 48% placebo	0.56 (95% CI 0.48 to 0.66)	5 (95% CI 4 to 6) over a mean time of 16 months

Adverse events were reported incompletely. The most common adverse events documented in continuation and maintenance phases were headache (weighted mean incidence 15.5%) and nausea (7.4%). Based on data pooled from 18 of the RCT's, loss to follow up due to adverse events was not statistically significantly different between antidepressant and placebo (relative risk=1.42, CI = 0.92 to 2.20).

The primary limitation of this review is the lack of studies designed to specifically answer our study question – the minimum duration of continued treatment to prevent relapse or recurrence. Only one study[44] randomized patients in remission to varying durations (14, 30 or 50 weeks) of continuation phase antidepressant or placebo. Relapse rates were significantly lower for patients on active treatment at 14 weeks (26% vs. 49%), and 38 weeks (9% vs. 23%) but not at 50 weeks (11% vs. 16%). Only 62 patients were randomized to 50 weeks treatment and the finding of no benefit is inconsistent with the overall body of evidence. A second limitation is incomplete descriptions of the study setting, recruitment approach and patient clinical and demographic characteristics. Careful descriptions of study populations, including risk factors for relapse would help decision makers apply these data. If patients included were at particularly high risk, then the estimates of baseline risk (from the placebo control groups) would not apply to patients with uncomplicated depression at low risk for relapse. Thus, the absolute benefit and number needed to treat (NNT) could be overstated.

Our search for additional RCT's identified three eligible studies published since the systematic review. The Prevention of Recurrent Episodes of Depression with Venlafaxine for Two Years (PREVENT) was a multi-phase, double-blind, placebo-controlled study of patients with recurrent MDD. Analyses from two phases of this larger study[37, 39] were relevant to KQ2. In the first phase,[37] participants who maintained a satisfactory response or clinical remission after acute phase and six months continuation phase treatment were randomized to 12-month maintenance treatment with venlafaxine ER or placebo. Venlafaxine ER was associated with a statistically significantly lower recurrence rate at 12-month follow-up (23.1% vs. 42.0%). The study had significantly higher loss to follow-up in the placebo group, which may have underestimated the difference between relapse rates. In the second phase[39] patients maintaining response at 12 months in phase 1 were re-randomized into a second 12 month course of venlafaxine ER or placebo. Failure to maintain response was defined as an increase in maintenance dose to 300mg/day or recurrence (HDRS-17 score > 12 and reduction of <= 50% from acute-phase baseline). Kaplan-Meier probability estimates for maintaining response across the combined 2 years of maintenance therapy were 67% for venlafaxine ER <= 225 mg/day and 41% for placebo (P =

0.007). This second report from the PREVENT study was of fair quality and did not report an analysis of patients lost to follow up in placebo or antidepressant groups, thus limiting applicability of its conclusions.

A good quality RCT[38] reported the results of a 24 week randomized controlled trial of escitalopram (10-20 mg per day) versus placebo in older adults who responded to a 12 week trial of open label escitalopram for treatment of a major depressive episode. The proportion of patients who relapsed within 24 weeks was significantly higher in the placebo group (33%; 50 patients) than in the escitalopram group (9%; 13 patients), (p<0.001). A small, fair quality RCT[36] reported the one-year follow up of 106 patients who had responded to 16 weeks of treatment with paroxetine, cognitive therapy, or behavioral activation. Of the 49 responders allocated randomly to either continued paroxetine treatment (n=28) or to placebo (n=21), relapse rates were 53% for antidepressant medication and 59% for placebo.

These additional studies support the findings of the systematic review. Continued treatment for 1 to 2 years after achieving partial- or full-remission with second-generation antidepressants decreases the risk of relapse or recurrence by almost 50%. Based on RCT's with some important limitations, generally consistent results and a precise estimate of effect, we grade the overall strength of evidence for this finding is moderate.

SUMMARY AND DISCUSSION

For KQ1, we only found studies addressing the responsiveness of the PHQ-9 and PHQ-2. In these few studies, there was a consistent association between PHQ-9 change scores and interview-based assessments of clinical status. The single study comparing the PHQ-9 and PHQ-2 showed comparable responsiveness. One study[34] included VA settings and is directly applicable to VA populations. In this study, a direct comparison of PHQ-9 to a longer questionnaire showed comparable responsiveness. Another study conducted relevant subgroup analyses with the German language version of the PHQ-9 and found similar responsiveness for important subgroups including men and women, and patients with comorbid medical conditions. A single study examined the minimum clinically important difference (MCID) and conservatively estimated this value as a 5 point change. This finding is consistent with other studies that use cross-sectional analyses to infer the MCID.[41] In summary, the PHQ-9 is the best validated instrument for identifying depressed patients in primary care [14-16]and for detecting clinically important response to treatment.

A recent literature synthesis [8] identified baseline and follow-up assessment of depression symptoms with a standardized scale as key features of effective depression care. The PHQ-9 appears well suited for this purpose and has been used in large VA evaluations of depression care.[45] Based on a single study conducted in Germany, the PHQ-2 appears responsive to change but only tracks two criterion symptoms and does not include an assessment of suicidal ideation. Based on this limited data and concerns about inadequate clinical data, the PHQ-2 alone cannot be recommended to monitor treatment response for clinical purposes. It may be useful for research studies when very brief instruments are needed. Our review was based in part on the assumption that questionnaires need to be brief to allow for both self-administration and interview administration in person or by telephone as is often done in integrated mental health-primary care models. Other, longer instruments may be preferred if the data collection burden can be eased through interactive voice response, web-based applications or scanable forms and the instrument has superior clinical content, better responsiveness or a better defined minimum clinically important difference. In addition, the response burden would need to be acceptable to patients.

Qualitative studies show that patients favor questionnaires to measure depression severity but general practitioners in the UK were cautious about the validity and utility of these measures and skeptical about the motives behind their introduction.[46] General practitioners specifically valued clinical judgment more than objective assessment. Practitioners were aware of the potential for manipulation of indicators for economic reasons. In the U.S.A., the PHQ-9 has been successfully implemented into primary care and psychiatric practices as part of quality improvement studies[47] and pragmatic clinical trials.[48, 49] These findings suggest that successful implementation of the PHQ-9 (or any other measure) will need to address attitudinal barriers and provide logistical support to integrate PHQ-9 administration into routine clinical processes.

For KQ2, the high quality systematic review[35] and 2 of the most recent relevant RCT's provide moderately strong evidence that continued antidepressant treatment decreases the risk of subsequent relapse for patients with MDD who achieve partial- or full-remission. The magnitude of risk reduction was similar for shorter- and longer-term trials and maintained for up to 2 years. The number needed to treat to prevent one relapse over a mean time of 8 or 16 months was 5. However, these trials do not directly answer our question about the minimum duration of continued antidepressant treatment since they report the average risk reduction over these time periods. In the single trial randomizing patients to differing durations of continuation treatment, the risk reduction was similar for 14 and 38 weeks but declined by 50 weeks. More studies utilizing this design in patients with various risks of relapse would better address the issue of minimum duration.

At the individual patient level, the decision for how long to continue antidepressant treatment should be based on effectiveness, adverse effects and patient preferences. These studies show clinically important risk reduction and adverse event rates similar to or slightly lower than acute phase treatment studies. A comprehensive review of adverse effects was beyond the scope of this study, but a careful evaluation of long-term adverse effects would be important to an accurate assessment of net benefit. Emerging evidence from observational studies suggest that newer antidepressants may increase the risk of osteoporosis[12, 13] or gastrointestinal bleeding in patients with concurrent non-steroidal anti-inflammatory drugs or low dose aspirin. Given the high rates of indicated aspirin use in the veteran population, a careful weighing of benefits and risks is needed and will depend in part on the patient's baseline risk of relapse or recurrence. As baseline risk of relapse increases, the absolute benefit increases. Since these studies appeared to enroll patients primarily from mental health settings, these patients may have been at higher risk than the average primary care patient with major depression. However two factors argue for applicability to primary care. First, the trials excluded patients with concurrent psychiatric conditions that may have increased the risk of relapse. Second, the large primary care based study by Unutzer et al.[50] included VA settings and found that almost three-quarters of patients with major depression had at least two prior episodes, a strong predictor of relapse risk. The current APA guidelines recommend at least 16-20 weeks of continuation treatment after remission is achieved and a judgment about maintenance treatment that is individually tailored to the patient. Other guidelines recommend longer treatment in patients at elevated risk. A key point and one that may require increased attention in primary care is need for a careful assessment of relapse risk when making the decision about continuing antidepressants beyond the acute and continuation phase treatment.

LIMITATIONS

Our review has a number of potential limitations. First, there are no validated search strategies to identify the literature for KQ1, increasing the risk that we may have missed relevant studies. Second, there were insufficient studies to do quantitative evaluations for publication bias or statistical heterogeneity. In addition, these types of studies are not typically included in clinical trials registries, further limiting our ability to detect publication bias. Third, we did not include studies that examined simple change in depression scores without a comparator to an interview-based measure of response. These studies could provide some, although less convincing evidence for responsiveness. Finally, the same author (Lowe) used three separate datasets from different study populations to conduct the relevant analyses. Replication by multiple investigators could increase confidence in the results.

For KQ2, the search strategy did not include foreign-language or articles published outside the Medline® database, potentially excluding relevant findings. However, the systematic review that was identified was recent, high quality, and addressed heterogeneity and publication bias. The systematic review looked to compare relapse rates for placebo and antidepressants during continuation and maintenance phase, but did not address directly the optimal duration of treatment. The two higher quality RCT's we identified found results consistent with the systematic review. Finally, we did not address first-generation antidepressants.

Conclusions

Table 7. Summary of Systematic Evidence Review by Key Question

KQ	Key Question	Type of Evidence	Quality of Evidence	Comments
1	Responsiveness of depression questionnaires	Observational	Moderate	PHQ-9 is responsive to change (mean change -11.2 to -6.7 for responders; standardized response mean -2.15 to -1.4)
2	Minimum duration of continued antidepressant treatment in patients achieving remission	RCT's	Moderate	Continued antidepressant treatment decreases the risk of relapse by 0.54 to 0.56 for up to two years (Number needed to treat = 5)

Determining the Responsiveness of Depression Questionnaires and Optimal Treatment Duration for Antidepressant Medications

Evidence-based Synthesis Program

FUTURE RESEARCH

Although moderately strong evidence shows the PHQ-9 is sensitive to change, studies that use receiver operating characteristic analysis to determine how well specific change scores classify patients into improved and unchanged or worse would be useful. These studies could help establish the minimum clinically important difference, which currently is based on limited data. Since data are limited in important subgroups (e.g., medical comorbidity, psychiatric comorbidity), studies evaluating responsiveness in key subgroups could also strengthen validity. Brief depression questionnaires, such as the PHQ-9, could be used in VA for performance measurement. Performance indicators could include: baseline administration at diagnosis (as an indicator of careful diagnostic assessment), administration longitudinally (as an indicator of careful follow-up), change scores or proportion achieving clinical response, or linked indicators that examine changes in treatment matched to changes in severity scores. Studies to examine the feasibility, acceptability to patients and clinicians, validity and impact on process of care and patient outcomes could help inform policy. If undertaken, these studies should include provisions for evaluating any unexpected consequences of introducing these measures into routine practice.

Although it is clear that continued antidepressant treatment beyond the acute phase decreases relapse, the optimal duration of treatment remains uncertain. Some clinical guidelines recommend that maintenance treatment duration should be customized based on risk factors for relapse, but the randomized trials we reviewed did not examine a risk factor based strategy. Future studies should carefully describe patient characteristics, such as number of prior depressive episodes that may predict relapse. These data would aid clinicians in applying these data and could help explain heterogeneity in treatment effects. Most importantly, analysis of a timeline for patients during continuation and maintenance phase would be most informative, documenting critical periods of increased relapse if they exist and measuring the balance between adverse effects and beneficial effects as patients stay on the antidepressant versus placebo treatment. It would also be informative to compare the different second-generation antidepressants, as well as compare first and second generation antidepressants.

Determining the Responsiveness of Depression Questionnaires and Optimal Treatment Duration for Antidepressant Medications

Evidence-based Synthesis Program

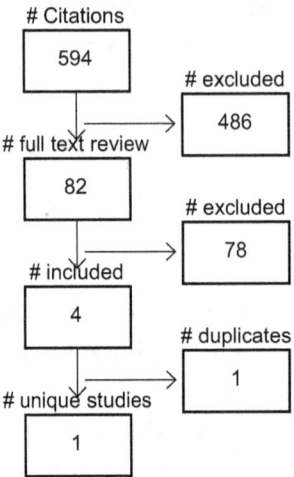

Figure 2. Key Question #1 Literature Flow

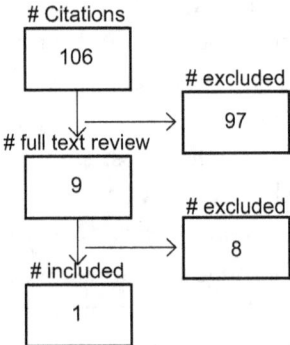

Figure 3. Key Question #2 Literature Flow

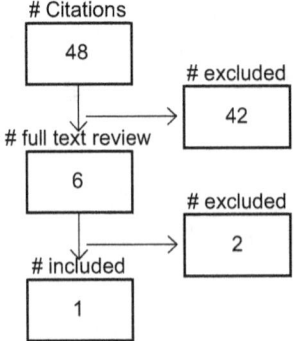

Figure 4. Key Question #2 Randomized Control Trials Literature Flow

APPENDIX A: SEARCH STRATEGIES

KEY QUESTION #1

Database: PubMed ® <1950 to February 2, 2009>

1	"Depressive Disorder, Major"[Mesh] OR (major AND depression)	32348
2	PHQ9 OR "Patient Health Questionnaire" OR "Beck Depression Inventory" OR BDI OR BDI-II OR GDS OR "Geriatric Depression Scale" OR SDDS-PC OR "symptom driven diagnostic system primary care" OR PRIMEMD OR "Primary care evaluation of mental disorders" OR DEPS OR "CESD" OR "CES-D" OR ("Center" AND Epidemiologic* AND Stud* AND Depression) OR "CESD-10"	11913
3	(change OR changes OR Improv* OR decreas*) AND (score OR scale* OR scores OR responsiv* OR sensitiv*)	447184
4	#1 AND #2 AND #3	522
5	(questionnaire OR psychometrics) AND ("Depressive Disorder, Major"[Mesh] OR (major AND depression)) AND (((responsiv*[tw] OR sensitiv*[tw]) AND (change[tw] OR changes[tw])) OR (clinical*[tw] AND important[tw] AND (change[tw] OR changes[tw])))	126
6	#4 OR #5	626
7	#6 Limits: Humans, English, All Adult: 19+ years	516

Database: PsychInfo <up to February 2, 2009>

1	major depression/	58084
2	major depression.tw.	16118
3	(PHQ9 or "Patient Health Questionnaire" or "Beck Depression Inventory" or BDI or BDI-II or GDS or "Geriatric Depression Scale" OR SDDS-PC or "symptom driven diagnostic system primary care" or PRIMEMD or "Primary care evaluation of mental disorders" or DEPS).tw.	9324
4	((change or changes or Improv* or decreas*) and (score or scale* or scores or responsiv* or sensitiv*)).tw.	82044
5	#1 or #2	61641
6	#3 and #4 and #5	893
7	limit 6 to (("followup study" or "longitudinal study" or "prospective study" or "systematic review") AND "adulthood age 18 yrs AND older" AND "peer-reviewed journal" AND English AND human)	157

KEY QUESTION #2, SYSTEMATIC REVIEWS

Database: PubMed ® <1950 to March 02, 2009>

1	("Depressive Disorder"[Mesh] OR "major depression")	63463
2	(antidepress* OR "Antidepressive Agents"[Mesh] OR "Antidepressive Agents "[Pharmacological Action])	114617
3	(recurrence[Mesh] OR relaps* OR recurren*)	410446
4	#1 AND #2 AND #3	2073
5	#4 AND systematic[sb]	106

KEY QUESTION #2, RANDOMIZED CONTROLLED TRIALS

Database: PubMed ® <1950 to March 01, 2009>

1	("Depressive Disorder"[Mesh] OR "major depression")	63463
2	(antidepress* OR "Antidepressive Agents"[Mesh] OR "Antidepressive Agents "[Pharmacological Action])	114617
3	(recurrence[Mesh] OR relaps* OR recurren*)	410446
4	(randomized controlled trial[Publication Type] OR (randomized[Title/Abstract] AND controlled[Title/Abstract] AND trial[Title/Abstract])	275051
5	#1 AND #2 AND #3 AND #4	428
6	Limits: Publication Date from 2007/01/01 to 2009/03/1, Humans, English, All Adult: 19+ years	48

APPENDIX B: FULL TEXT EXCLUSIONS

Inclusion Criteria for Key Question #1, Assessment Tools Responsive to Change

1. One of the specified instruments (PHQ-9, Beck Fast Screen, CESD-10, GDS-15, SDDS-PC, DEPS, PRIME MD)
2. Adults with depressive disorder: outpatient setting
3. Comparator: Comparison to an interview-based instrument
4. Study Design: Longitudinal
5. Study Design: Sample > 50
6. English language article

Author & Ref #	General Exclusion Criteria*					
	NOT 1.	NOT 2.	NOT 3.	NOT 4.	NOT 5.	NOT 6.
Ahava, 1998[51]	X					
Adler, 2004[52]			X			
Allard, 2004[53]	X					
Altamura, 1989[54]	X					
Amsterdam, 2008[55]		X				
Babyak, 2000[56]	X					
Baldwin, 2008[57]	X					
Barbosa, 2003[58]	X					
Berkman, 2003[59]	X					
Berlim, 2005[60]						X
Berlim, 2007[61]						X
Boyer, 1998[62]	X					
Brody, 2006[63]			X			
Brown, 2000[64]	X					
Brown, 2005[65]	X					
Cassidy, 2005[66]					X	
Casten, 2000[67]		X				
Chen, 2006[68]						X
Conradi, 2007[69]	X					
Cook,1999[70]					X	
Corney, 2005[71]			X			
Coulehan, 1997[72]	X					
Dalton, 2000[73]					X	
Davies, 2003[74]					X	
DeBattista, 2003[75]					X	
Dori, 1999[76]	X					

Author & Ref #	General Exclusion Criteria*					
	NOT 1.	NOT 2.	NOT 3.	NOT 4.	NOT 5.	NOT 6.
Dubovsky, 2001[77]					X	
Dunner, 1987[78]	X					
Einarson, 2004[79]	X					
Fava, 1999[80]					X	
Fawcett, 1987[81]	X					
George, 1999[82]	X					
George, 2008[83]	X					
Goodnick, 1997[84]					X	
Goodnick, 1998[85]	X					
Judd, 2004[86]	X					
Kates, 2002[87]	X					
Koivumaa-Honkanen, 2008[88]	X					
Koran, 1995[89]	X					
Kroenke, 2006[90]	X					
Lesperance, 2007[91]	X					
Lett, 2007[92]	X					
Levitt, 1999[93]					X	
Liebowitz, 2007[94]	X					
Lustman, 1998[95]			X			
Lustman, 2000[96]	X					
Lydiard, 1997[97]	X					
Mazeh, 2007[98]					X	
McIntyre, 2005[99]	X					
Mohamed, 2006[100]	X					
Mulrow, 1998[101]	X					
Mynors-Wallis, 2000[102]	X					
Patkar, 2006[103]	X					
Perez, 1999[104]	X					
Picardi, 2005[105]		X				
Pollock, 1989[106]		X				
Posternak, 2001[107]	X					
Proudfoot, 2003[108]			X			
Pyne, 2002[109]		X				
Quilty, 2008[110]	X					
Raskin, 2003[111]	X					
Raskin, 2007[112]	X					
Rollman, 2002[113]	X					

Author & Ref #	General Exclusion Criteria*					
	NOT 1.	NOT 2.	NOT 3.	NOT 4.	NOT 5.	NOT 6.
Rush, 2005[114]	X					
Rutherford, 2007[115]						X
Salkovskis, 2006[116]	X					
Shelton, 2001[117]	X					
Singh, 2001[118]						X
Skevington, 2001[119]	X					
Spalletta, 2002[120]						X
Stark, 1985[121]			X			
Szegedi, 2005[122]	X					
Thase, 1997[123]	X					
Trivedi, 2004[124]	X					
Tutty, 2000[125]	X					
van Gurp, 2002[126]	X					
van Marwijk, 2008[127]			X			
Vinkers, 2004[128]		X				
Wade, 2008[129]	X					
Wise, 2007[130]	X					

Items in the table (e.g. Not 1) correspond to the inclusion criteria listed above the table

Inclusion Criteria for Key Question #2, Systematic Reviews

1. Systematic review evaluating anti-depressant vs. placebo. A systematic review contains a methods section with search strategy and approach to synthesizing the data
2. Patients: Adults with major depressive disorder who have remitted or improved substantially with anti-depressant medication, English language article
3. Outcome: Relapse/recurrence

Author & Ref #	General Exclusion Criteria*		
	NOT 1.	NOT 2.	NOT 3.
Bauer 2009[131]			X
Gartlehener 2008[132]			X
Quaseem 2008[133]	X		
Anderson 2008[134]	X		
Papakostas 2007[135]			X
Furukawa 2007[136]	X		
Zimmerman 2007[137]			X
Lam 2004[138]	X		

Items in the table (e.g. Not 1) correspond to the inclusion criteria listed above the table*

Inclusion Criteria for Key Question #2, Randomized Controlled Trials

1. Study Design: Randomized Controlled Trial
2. Patients: Adults
3. Outcome: Relapse/recurrence
4. Compares anti-depressant vs. placebo
5. Patients: Adults with major depressive disorder who have remitted or improved substantially with anti-depressant medication
6. English language article

Author & Ref #	General Exclusion Criteria*					
	NOT 1.	NOT 2.	NOT 3.	NOT 4.	NOT 5.	NOT 6.
Dombrovski 2008[139]					X	
Keller 2007[140]				X		

*Items in the table (e.g. Not 1) correspond to the inclusion criteria listed above the table

APPENDIX C: QUALITY RATINGS

QUALITY RATING FOR KEY QUESTION #1, ASSESSMENT TOOLS RESPONSIVE TO CHANGE

Was the criterion standard applied and interpreted blinded to the results of the depression questionnaire?

Was the depression questionnaire applied and interpreted blinded to the results of the criterion standard?

Was the interview-based criterion standard a validated measure of depression severity?

Did follow-up of the enrolled sample exceed 80%?

Was the analysis appropriate to the study question?

Was the study funded by the pharmaceutical industry?

Was a conflict of interest disclosure given? If given, was there a potential conflict of interest?

QUALITY RATING FOR KEY QUESTION #2, SYSTEMATIC REVIEWS

Was a focused clinical question clearly stated?

Was the search for relevant studies detailed and exhaustive?

Were inclusion/exclusion criteria clearly defined and appropriate?

Were primary studies evaluated for quality and appropriateness?

Were assessments of studies reproducible?

Were analyses conducted to measure variability in effect?

Were differences in how outcomes were reported and analyzed across studies were taken into consideration?

Was publication bias assessed?

Were clinically important outcomes (harms and benefits) reported?

Were the conclusions supported by the data presented?

QUALITY RATING FOR KEY QUESTION #2, RANDOMIZED CONTROLLED TRIALS

Were the groups similar at baseline in terms of baseline characteristics and prognostic factors?

Were depression outcomes assessed using a valid methodology and criteria?

Were subjects and providers blind to the intervention/exposure status of participants?

Were outcome assessors blind to exposure/intervention status?

Were incomplete outcome data adequately addressed?

Was there an important differential loss to follow-up between the compared groups (defined as $\geq$ 10%)?

Was there an overall high loss to follow-up ($\geq$ 20% for studies <12 months and $\geq$ 30% for studies of 12 month or longer duration)

Was there a conflict of interest?

Were the methods used for randomization adequate?

Was allocation concealment adequate?

APPENDIX D: PEER REVIEW

Question: Are the objectives, scope, and methods for this review clearly described?		
Reviewer	**Comment**	**Reply**
1	YES. The objectives, scope were very clear and appropriate. The methods were transparent and appropriately rigorous for a best evidence review, even though the types of studies sought to answer KQ1 and KQ2 were very different. It was helpful to have all of the information on search strategies, inclusion/exclusion criteria and data extraction in the appendices.	Acknowledged
2	The inclusion and exclusion criteria for Key Question 1 greatly diminish the synthesis's scope. Given this limitation, I know of no additional studies that should have been included in the review for Key Question 1 or 2. In general, the Synthesis needs a strong editing (e.g. ensuring consistency in abbreviations, defining abbreviations before applying them, correcting punctuation and formatting) In addition, there were several places within the synthesis where this reviewer could not understand the meaning of a sentence. Specifically: • Page 8, line 11-12 – "For the finding that the MCID is 5" would be best to define this as the Mean Change in Depression Score for MDD • Page 16, line 11 – "the similarity of groups similar at baseline" • Page 25, line 2 – "the number needed"…(number of what?) • The Evidence Tables 1-5 are very difficult to read because of inconsistent formatting and text layout.	The inclusion/exclusion criteria were developed with the stakeholders to focus on the questions of interest. Editing has been completed to ensure consistency These sentences have been edited to clarify the meaning. We did not find the Page 25, line 2 reference; on page 26 we state the "number needed to treat to prevent one relapse…"
3	Yes, all of these aspects are clearly described.	Acknowledged
4	a) Objectives are clearly defined. b) Scope is also clearly defined, with the exception that the assessment tools that are surveyed are those immediately referable to depressive disorders and their symptoms (i.e., disease-specific). One could also perceive quality of life, functional capacities, health services utilization and costs as relevant outcomes. I agree with focusing on disease-specific assessment, and this is clear as the manuscript goes on, but I would make it absolutely clear up front so as to frame the boundaries of this review explicitly. c) Methods are clearly defined.	Acknowledged Edits made to clarify that focus is limited to depression symptom questionnaires Acknowledged

Question: Is there any indication of bias in our synthesis of the evidence?		
Reviewer	**Comment**	**Reply**
1	NO. Appropriate precautions were used to minimize bias including 1) having 2 researchers review the titles and/or abstracts of articles for potential inclusion, 2) having 1-2 reviewers over-read the data abstraction forms to assure accurate abstraction, 3) using well known criteria to assess the quality of the studies that included items about funding source and conflict of interest (Appendix C) and strength of evidence (GRADE), 4) providing readers with enough detail to assure transparency, and 5) including comments from outsider reviewers in an Appendix.	Acknowledged
2	It was not clear how this group of authors was selected to conduct the evidence synthesis. Was this a competitive application or were the authors selected based on their willingness to conduct the synthesis, their expertise in the area of study, or other factors?	This has been addressed in the topic refinement section
3	No, there is no indication of bias	Acknowledged
4	No	Acknowledged

Question: Are there any studies on responsiveness of depression questionnaires or relapse prevention trials related to this report that we have overlooked?		
Reviewer	**Comment**	**Reply**
1	NO. These are difficult studies to do well and get funded appropriately since they require a diagnostic interview as a reference standard (KQ1) and have a long follow-up period (KQ2). I was not surprised that few studies were found.	Acknowledged
2	None	
3	No, there are no responsiveness studies missed to include in the analysis. However, in the discussion of results, the authors refer to a UK qualitative study suggesting clinicians are skeptical of depression questionnaires. If this study is cited, the authors should also cite two recent studies showing US primary care physicians (Nease et al, 2008) and psychiatrists (Duffy et al) found the PHQ-9 clinically useful and continued to use. Also, the authors did not include the 10-item CES-D short-form (Andresen et al, 1994). There are probably no studies testing its responsiveness, but I mention it simply because it does fall within the authors' 10-item inclusion criteria for brief measures. • Nease DE, Nutting PA, Dickinson WP, Bonham AJ, Graham DG, Gallagher KM, Main DS. Inducing sustainable improvement in depression care in primary care practices. Joint Commission Journal on Quality and Patient Safety 2008;34:247-255. • Duffy FF, Chung H, Trivedi M, Rae DS, Regier DA, Katzelnick DJ. Systematic use of patient-rated depression severity monitoring: is it helpful and feasible in clinical psychiatry? Psychiatric Services 2008;59:1148–1154. • Andresen EM, Malmgren JA, Carter WB, Patrick DL. Screening for depression in well older adults: evaluation of a short form of the CES-D (Center for Epidemiologic Studies Depression Scale). Am J Prev Med. 1994; 10: 77–84.	The discussion has been revised and the additional studies referenced The CESD-10 was not excluded but our search did not include terms specific to this instrument. We have updated the search and results. 49 additional citations were identified but none met eligibility criteria
4	None that meet the defined criteria, to my knowledge	Acknowledged

Question: Please write additional suggestions or additional comments below for this report. If applicable, please indicate the page and line numbers from the draft report.		
Reviewer	**Comment**	**Reply**
1	The target audience for this report includes administrators and policy makers. They would benefit from a conclusion section at the end of the Executive Summary that simply stated the conclusions followed by quality of the evidence supporting the conclusion. This could even be 2 bullet points. Administrators and policy makers are likely to start with this bottom line and read backwards if they need more detail. For example, you could use lines 14-16 on page 24, lines 11-15 on page 23, and lines 44-46 and 1-4 on pages 24 and 25 after editing them. For KQ2, it helps to have both the RR and NNT.	We have followed this suggestion
	The results section in the Executive Summary was difficult to follow for KQ1, lines 31-43, page 7. The methods paragraph describes the standardized response mean (SRM) then the results start with the mean change score. I would list the mean change score and SRM for 3 months, then for 6 months. Although you save words in the current version, it is harder to read. Also in line 41 define the abbreviation MCID since you use it later.	We have followed this suggestion
	Figure 1 on page 13 is difficult to read in its current size. It would be good if it could be enlarged.	The figure has been enlarged
	In Table 7 on page 26, it would be helpful to include some data in the comments section after the summary comment, e.g., mean change score expected of responders. Also, I would include the NNT with the RR.	We have followed this suggestion
	Appendix B is important to document why studies were excluded/include. Using "not 1," "not 2," etc is a bit confusing, but I could not think of a better way to concisely describe these criteria for the table headers.	Modified to improve clarity
	In Appendix C, page 37, line 30 has a typo. I think it should read "... evaluated for quality and appropriateness?"	Thank you. Typo corrected
	The evidence tables are dense, but the details are important for transparency.	Acknowledged

| 2 | **Key Question 1**
In general, this reviewer felt that Key Question 1 was not an "assessment of tools that were responsive to change", but rather a review of the PHQ-9's (and at times the PHQ-2's) responsiveness to change. This apparent bias first appears in the background section in which the synthesis first author's work (reference 15) concluded that the PHQ-9 had better performance characteristics and gave more information for depression diagnosis than other instruments. Thus, from the very beginning, this reviewer was confused on why Key Question 1 was requested for a synthesis review.

Given these issues, the background on Depression Questionnaires either 1) needs to be expanded to describe the 7 other questionnaires that have < 10 items, or 2) for the sake of transparency, the background section should clearly state in the text that the work that identified the PHQ-9 as the optimal self reported primary care depression measure was conducted by the first author of this synthesis.

The fact that the primary manuscripts reviewed for Key Question 1 (references 29-32) were all conducted by the same first author (Lowe) should be noted in the limitations.

Since the authors note that there has been no work to date measuring responsiveness to change in instruments was for the PHQ-9 and was applied in a population greater than age 60, the Future Research section should also call for additional studies to identify whether or not the PHQ-9 (and other measures) respond to change in younger populations.

Key Question 2
Given that the number of prior episodes is a major risk for relapse, did any of the RCT's reviewed for Key Question 2 address this issue? Though this is alluded to on page 22, lines 17-20, it should be more clearly stated. | We have attempted to strengthen the message that we searched for ALL feasible instruments, but only found data for the PHQ. The background has been modified to briefly describe the eligible questionnaires.

Discussion has been updated to note this issue.

No change; the PHQ9 has been evaluated in mid-life and older adults

The number of prior depressive episodes was not systematically reported in the trials |
| 3 | Page 6, lines 17-36: In paragraph, authors state "Clinical guidelines recommend continuation treatment for 4-6 months … However, clinical guidelines for longer-term maintenance phase treatment are more variable and performance indicators (e.g., HEDIS) do not address maintenance phase treatment." But Key Question #2 is: "What is the minimum duration of continuation phase treatment to decrease risk of relapse?" Continuation (1st 4-9 months after remission) and maintenance (long-term treatment after continuation) phases of treatment have distinct meanings in some guidelines, and the authors' going back and forth between these 2 terms (and in other places the vaguer phrase "long-term treatment" leaves the reader confused whether their review is focused on evidence for continuation phase treatment, maintenance phase, or both. Please clarify for reader.

Page 8, Lines 31-46: This section clarifies the answer to the question above (i.e., this review looks at both continuation and maintenance treatment) – this should be clarified on p. 6 | This comment and the following comment have been addressed in the revision. The background on page 6 clarifies that the review addressed continuation and maintenance phase treatment

As above |

Page 14, Lines 36-37: There is a short-form of the CES-D (10 items). The reference is provided under #3 above. The authors might note why this was not included in their search.	Previously addressed
Page 15, Lines 7-8: The authors might add to their parenthetical examples of measures longer than 10 items the Inventory for Depressive Symptoms (since it was used in the landmark STAR*D trial where 40% of patients were from primary care) and the CES-D.	This recommendation was followed
Page 18, Lines 7-9: The authors state: "In addition the study team included a biostatistician from Pfizer, and Pfizer funded the current study and the PHQ-9 development, suggesting a potential conflict of interest." However, unlike drugs sold for profit, the PHQ-9 always has been made available free of charge. Thus, the potential conflict of interest is much weaker than if drug trials were being analyzed.	This is a valid point about the availability free of charge. However, potential COI still exists as increased identification of depression may increase sales or related for-profit products. No change
Page 24, Lines 35-42: The authors state: "Qualitative studies show that patients favor questionnaires to measure depression severity but general practitioners in the UK were cautious about the validity and utility of these measures and skeptical about the motives behind their introduction. General practitioners specifically valued clinical judgment more than objective assessment. Practitioners were aware of the potential for manipulation of indicators for economic reasons. If these findings hold true for VA clinicians, these barriers would need to be addressed for successful implementation of the PHQ-9 (or any other measure) for routine monitoring." However, two recent studies in the US showed good uptake of the PHQ-9 by primary care physicians (Nease et al 2008) and psychiatry (Duffy et al 2008).	Previously addressed

Question: Recommendations for future ESP topical areas of interest or programmatic comments may also be included at the end of this section.

Reviewer	Comment	Reply
1	Topics: 1. Treatment of chronic obstructive pulmonary disease 2. Palliative chemotherapy for lung, colon, and possibly other cancers Programmatic Comments: 1. Translating evidence syntheses into policy and organizational decisions will be a difficult step. I assume the ESPs are linked to OQP, but there should be outreach to VISNs and medical centers.	Acknowledged Acknowledged
2	None	
3	None at this time	
4	If feasible, a review of evidence-based methods and data on suicide risk evaluation in primary care settings would be helpful	Acknowledged

Determining the Responsiveness of Depression Questionnaires and
Optimal Treatment Duration for Antidepressant Medications

Evidence-based Synthesis Program

APPENDIX E: EVIDENCE TABLES

Evidence Table 1. Key Question #2 Systematic Review, Hansen, 2008[35]

Studies	Study Characteristics / Study Designs	Patient Characteristics	Outcomes Assessed	Relative risks/other summary effect measures	Comments / Quality Rating
Doogan & Caillard, 1992[141] Feiger, 1999[142] Gelenberg, 2003[143] Gilaberte, 2001[144] Hochstrasser, 2001[145] Keller, 1998[146] Klysner, 2002[147] Kornstein, 2006[42] Lepine, 2004[43] Lustman, 2006[148] Montgomery, 1993[149] Montgomery, 2004[150] Montgomery & Dunbar, 1993[151] Rapaport, 2004 [not found] Reimherr, 1998[44] Reynolds, 2006[152] Robert & Montgomery, 1995[153] Schmidt, 2000[154] Simon, 2004[155] Terra & Montgomery, 1998[156] Thase, 2001[157] Weihs, 2002[158] Wilson, 2003[159]	**No. of studies: 23** placebo controlled RCT **Study countries:** Most included US Many in UK, France, & Europe Several multinational **Study intervention:** Second-generation antidepressant: bupropion, citalopram, duloxetine, escitalopram, fluoxetine, fluvoxamine, mirtazapine, nefazodone, paroxetine, sertraline, trazodone, venlafaxine **Clinical settings (22/23 articles):** Mixed settings: 4 "Outpatient": 12 Not Given: 6 VA: 0 Civilian: 22	**Total no. of patients:** 8241 **Age:** Mean age range generally 40-50. Two trials w/ range 65-87 **Gender:** Most >60% female Many >65% female **Depressive Disorder:** 26 required MDD diagnosis, 1 required only QIDS-C-16 > 5. **Severity of initial symptoms:** Many used HDRS. Some had requirement for # episodes. **Race/ethnicity:** NG **Exclusion:** Use of other psychotropics, presence of comorbid psychiatric or medical disease most common	**Relapse definition:** most used increase in HAM-D or MADRS above predefined cutoff pt. Some added clinical criteria. **Treatment duration (after acute phase):** Continuation: 14-72 weeks Maintenance: 36-100 weeks. 12 trials: f/up <1yr (re-defined as continuation) 11 trials: f/up 1+ yr (re-defined as maintenance) **Outcomes:** 1) Continuation phase relapse rate compared to placebo 2) Maintenance phase recurrence rate compared to placebo **Other Outcomes:** 4) Rates of adverse events 5) Rates of loss to f/up attributed to adverse events	Relapse re-defined as relapse w/in 1 yr continuation Recurrence re-defined as relapse w/in 1 yr maintenance **Outcomes:** 1) Unadjusted frequency of relapse was 22% active treatment, 42% placebo 2) Unadjusted frequency of recurrence was 26% for active treatment, 48% placebo **Other Outcomes:** 3) Adverse events rates given for individual studies when reported (compared w/ acute-phase studies, relative incidence of most common adverse events was lower) 5) Loss to f/up attributed to adverse events was 7% for active treatment and 4% for placebo (did not report significance)	**Comments:** -In meta-regression, duration of follow-up did not impact effect size -Authors reported fair quality of studies included -Moderate grade evidence **Quality Rating:** high Focused clinical question? Yes Detailed & exhaustive search? Yes Inclusion/exclusion criteria clearly defined & appropriate? Yes Studies evaluated for quality & appropriately? Yes Assessments of studies reproducible? Yes Measured variability in effect? Yes Differences in how outcomes were reported and analyzed across studies considered? Yes Publication bias assessed? Yes, Clinically important outcomes (harms & benefits) reported? Yes Conclusions supported by data presented? Yes

Determining the Responsiveness of Depression Questionnaires and
Optimal Treatment Duration for Antidepressant Medications

Evidence-based Synthesis Program

Evidence Table 2. Key Question #2 Randomized Controlled Trials

Study Characteristics	Research Objective Duration Study Design	Patient Baseline Characteristics	Inclusion/Exclusion Criteria	Outcome Results	Adverse Events (%)	Analysis Quality Rating
Author: Kocsis et al., 2007[37] **Country and Setting:** United States Outpatient **Funding:** Wyeth (manufacturer of venlafaxine)	**Research Objective:** To compare time to recurrence of depression with venlafaxine ER versus placebo **Duration of Study:** 12-month maintenance phase for venlafaxine ER responders **Study Design:** Randomized Placebo controlled **Overall Total N:** 258 (randomized) **Intervention:** Group 1: Venlafaxine ER 75-300 mg daily Group 2: Placebo	**Mean Age:** Venlafaxine ER 42.0 Placebo 42.6 **Sex (% female):** Venlafaxine ER 69% Placebo 67% **Race (% white):** Venlafaxine ER 81% Placebo 88% **Baseline (HDRS):** Venlafaxine ER 4.3 Placebo 4.9	**Inclusion Criteria:** • ≥ 18 years old • MDD by DSM-IV • Depression symptoms for ≥ 1 month • ≥3 prior depressive episodes, 2 in the past 5 years • Two months between episodes • HDRS-17 score ≥ 20 at screening and ≥18 at randomization • Response or remission of intake episode at end of continuation phase **Exclusion Criteria:** • Failed trial of study medications • Treatment resistant, defined as failure of three med trials, ECT, or psychotherapy • Hypersensitivity to study medications • Alcohol or illicit drug use within 6 months • Seizure disorder • Other serious medical diseases • Other mental illnesses • Pregnant or lactating • ECT within 3 months • Fluoxetine or MAO-I within 30 days • Other antidepressant within 14 days • Any other psychotropic drug 7 days	**Venlafaxine ER was associated with significantly lower risk of recurrence in comparison to placebo.** **Probability of recurrence:** **Month 6:** Venlafaxine ER: 18.8% Placebo: 28.4% **Month 12:** Venlafaxine ER: 23.1% Placebo: 42%	**Headache:** Venlafaxine ER 25 Placebo 24 **Upper Respiratory Infection:** Venlafaxine ER 17 Placebo 12 **Dry Mouth:** Venlafaxine ER 15 Placebo 11 **Insomnia:** Venlafaxine ER 14 Placebo 13 **Sweating:** Venlafaxine ER 14 Placebo 12 **Weight Gain:** Venlafaxine ER 12 Placebo 7 **Dizziness:** Venlafaxine ER 11 Placebo 21 **Nausea:** Venlafaxine ER 11 Placebo 10 **Sexual Problems:** Venlafaxine ER 11 Placebo 7	**Overall Attrition Rate:** Venlafaxine = 50% Placebo = 73% ($p<.001$) **ITT Analysis:** Yes **Quality Rating: fair?** Grps similar at baseline? Yes Outcomes used valid methodology & criteria? Yes, HDRS-17 Subjects & providers blind to intervention status of participants? Yes Outcome assessors blind? Yes Incomplete outcome data adequately addressed? Yes, ITT >10% differential loss to f/up between grps? Yes Overall >30% loss to f/up? Yes, 40% Conflict of interest? Funded by venlafaxine manufacturer Adequate randomization methods? NG Allocation concealment adequate? NG

Determining the Responsiveness of Depression Questionnaires and
Optimal Treatment Duration for Antidepressant Medications

Evidence-based Synthesis Program

Evidence Table 3. Key Question #2 Randomized Controlled Trials

Study Characteristics	Research Objective Duration Study Design	Patient Baseline Characteristics	Inclusion/Exclusion Criteria	Outcome Results	Adverse Effects	Analysis Quality Rating
Author: Kornstein et al., 2008[39] **Country and Setting:** United States Outpatient **Funding:** Wyeth (manufacturer of venlafaxine)	**Research Objective:** Evaluate the long-term efficacy of venlafaxine ER =< 225mg/day in patients with recurrent MDD **Duration of Study:** Two years for venlafaxine ER responders **Study Design:** Randomized Placebo controlled **Overall Total N:** 114 **Intervention:** Group 1: Continue venlafaxine ER 75-225mg/day Group 2: Placebo	**Mean Age:** Venlafaxine ER 41 Placebo 43.1 **Sex (% female):** Venlafaxine ER 73 Placebo 63 **Race (% white):** NG **Baseline (HDRS)** Venlafaxine 3.2 Placebo 4.5	**Inclusion Criteria:** • ≥18 years old • MDD by DSM-IV • Depression symptoms for ≥ 1 month • ≥ 3 prior depressive episodes, 2 in the past 5 years • Two months between episodes • HDRS-17 score ≥20 at screening and ≥18 at randomization • Response or remission of intake episode at end of continuation phase **Exclusion Criteria:** • Failed trial of study medications • Treatment resistant, defined as failure of three med trials, ECT, or psychotherapy • Hypersensitivity to study medications • Alcohol or illicit drug use within 6 months • Seizure Disorder • Others serious medical diseases • Other mental illnesses • Pregnant or Lactating • ECT within 3 months • Fluoxetine or MAO-I within 30 days • Other antidepressant within 14 days • Any other psychotropic drug 7 days	**Kaplan-Meier probability estimate for not experiencing recurrence OR increasing dose to 300mg/day:** **67% for venlafaxine ER =< 225 mg** **41% for placebo** NNT of 4.5 Estimated probability of not having recurrence greater in venlafaxine ER group vs. placebo (76% versus 58%) but did not reach level of statistical significance	Not reported	**Overall Attrition Rate:** NG **ITT Analysis:** Not done **Quality Rating: fair or poor?** Grps similar at baseline? Yes Outcomes used valid methodology & criteria? Partial, HDRS-17 & dose increase of antidepressant Subjects & providers blind to intervention status of participants? Yes Outcome assessors blind? Yes Incomplete outcome data adequately addressed? No, reasons not reported >10% differential loss to f/up between grps? No Overall >30% loss to f/up? No Conflict of interest? Funded by venlafaxine manufacturer Adequate randomization methods? NG Allocation concealment adequate? NG

40

Determining the responsiveness of Depression Questionnaires and
Optimal Treatment Duration for Antidepressant Medications

Evidence-based Synthesis Program

Evidence Table 4. Key Question #2 Randomized Controlled Trials

Study Characteristics	Research Objective Duration Study Design	Patient Baseline Characteristics	Inclusion/Exclusion Criteria	Outcome Results	Adverse Events (%)	Analysis Quality Rating
Author: Gorwood et al., 2007[38] **Country and Setting:** 7 European countries Outpatient **Funding:** H. Lundbeck A/S (manufacturer of escitalopram)	**Research Objective:** To test the hypothesis that fewer older patients will relapse on escitalopram compared with placebo **Duration of Study:** 24 week maintenance phase for escitalopram responders after 12 weeks of open label treatment **Study Design:** Randomized Placebo controlled **Overall Total N:** 305 (randomized) **Intervention:** Group 1: escitalopram 10-20 mg/day Group 2: placebo	**Mean Age:** Escitalopram 73 Placebo 72 **Sex (% female):** Escitalopram 78% Placebo 79% **Race (% white):** Escitalopram 99.7% Placebo 100% **Baseline (MADRS):** Escitalopram 5.1 Placebo 5.1	**Inclusion Criteria:** • >= 65 years old • MDD by MINI • Response to a 12 week trial of escitalopram • MADRS score >= 22 • Duration of t index episode of at least 4 weeks • MMSE score >= 24 **Exclusion Criteria:** • Current or past history of manic or hypomanic episode, psychotic disorder (including MDD with psychotic features), MR, or mental disorders resulting from a general medical condition • Any substance abuse disorder, presence or history of a clinically significant neurologic disorder, neurodegenerative disorder, and any personality disorder. • Significant suicide risk • Recent receipt prior to screening of the following treatments: ☐ antipsychotic drugs, ECT, lithium, carbamazepine, valproate, or valpromide ☐ antidepressants, benzodiazepines, non-benzodiazepine anxiolytics or hypnotics (other than zolpidem, zopiclone, or zaleplon); serotonin agonists (for example, triptans), psychotherapy ☐ hypersensitivity to citalopram and/or escitalopram ☐ resistance to two trials of antidepressants or resistance to citalopram or escitalopram	**Escitalopram was four times as effective as placebo in preventing relapse over 24 weeks in older patients with MDD who had achieved full remission** **Percentage who relapsed:** Escitalopram: 9% (13 patients) Placebo: 33% (50 patients)	**Any adverse event:** Escitalopram 35.3 Placebo 34.9 **Diarrhea:** Escitalopram 3.3 Placebo 2.6 **Dizziness:** Escitalopram 4.6 Placebo 3.3 **Nausea:** Escitalopram 0 Placebo 0 **Headache:** Escitalopram 2.6 Placebo 3.3	**Overall Attrition Rate:** Escitalopram = 15% Placebo = 8.5% (excluding relapsers) **ITT Analysis:** Yes **Quality Rating:** Grps similar at baseline? Yes Outcomes used valid methodology & criteria? Yes, MADRS Subjects & providers blind to intervention status of participants? Yes Outcome assessors blind? Yes Incomplete outcome data adequately addressed? Yes, ITT >10% differential loss to f/up between grps? No Overall >30% loss to f/up? No Conflict of interest? Funded by escitalopram manufacturer Adequate randomization methods? Yes Allocation concealment adequate? Yes

41

Determining the Responsiveness of Depression Questionnaires and
Optimal Treatment Duration for Antidepressant Medications

Evidence-based Synthesis Program

Evidence Table 5. Key Question #2 Randomized Controlled Trials

Study Characteristics	Research Objective Duration Study Design	Patient Baseline Characteristics	Inclusion/Exclusion Criteria	Outcome Results	Adverse Events (%)	Analysis Quality Rating
Author: Dobson et al., 2008[36] **Country and Setting:** United States Outpatient **Funding:** NIMH	**Research Objective:** To compare relapse rates among prior behavioral activation, prior cognitive therapy, and antidepressant medication (ADM) to placebo **Duration of Study:** 2 years of follow up after 16 week acute phase treatment. Pts were all withdrawn from ADM after 1 year. **Study Design:** Randomized Placebo controlled **Overall Total N:** 106 (randomized) **Intervention:** Group 1: paroxetine (28) Group 2: placebo (21)	Baseline characteristics of those randomized to ADM and placebo in the maintenance phase were not separately reported. **For all subjects randomized to AMD or placebo:** Female 78.2% Caucasian 80.0% Minority 20.0% Married 36.3% Have children 43.6% College education 63.8%	**Inclusion Criteria:** • response to acute phase treatment for depression with 16 weeks of paroxetine • diagnosis of MDD for index episode on the basis of diagnostic interviews • 20 or above on the Beck Depression Inventory II and scores of 14 or above on the 17-item version of the HDRS **Exclusion Criteria:** Not explicitly stated in this report	**Rates of relapse** after 1 year follow up from Cox regression analysis: paroxetine: 53% placebo: 59% (not statistically significantly different)	Not reported	**Overall Attrition Rate:** ADM = 7% Placebo = 19% **ITT Analysis:** Unclear **Quality Rating: Poor - Fair?** Grps similar at baseline? NG Outcomes used valid methodology & criteria? Yes, HRSD Subjects & providers blind to intervention status of participants? Yes Outcome assessors blind? Yes Incomplete outcome data adequately addressed? No, reasons not reported >10% differential loss to f/up between grps? Yes Overall >30% loss to f/up? No Conflict of interest? No, funded by NIMH Adequate randomization methods? Yes Allocation concealment adequate? Yes

REFERENCES (TEXT AND APPENDICES)

1. Murray, C.J. and A.D. Lopez, *Alternative projections of mortality and disability by cause 1990-2020: Global Burden of Disease Study.* Lancet, 1997. 349(9064): p. 1498-504.

2. Katon, W. and H. Schulberg, *Epidemiology of depression in primary care.* Gen Hosp Psychiatry, 1992. 14(4): p. 237-47.

3. Ormel, J., et al., *Recognition, management, and course of anxiety and depression in general practice.* Arch Gen Psychiatry, 1991. 48(8): p. 700-6.

4. Simon, G.E. and M. VonKorff, *Recognition, management, and outcomes of depression in primary care.* Archives of Family Medicine, 1995. 4(2): p. 99-105.

5. Gilbody, S., et al., *Collaborative cares for depression: a cumulative meta-analysis and review of longer-term outcomes.* Arch Intern Med, 2006. 166(21): p. 2314-21.

6. Gilbody, S., P. Bower, and P. Whitty, *Costs and consequences of enhanced primary care for depression: systematic review of randomized economic evaluations.* Br J Psychiatry, 2006. 189: p. 297-308.

7. Williams, J.W., Jr., et al., *Systematic review of multifaceted interventions to improve depression care.* Gen Hosp Psychiatry, 2007. 29(2): p. 91-116.

8. Rubenstein, L.V., et al., *Determining key features of effective depression interventions.*, V.A.H.S.R.D.S.E.-B.S. Program, Editor. 2009: Washington, DC.

9. Anonymous, *Depression: Management in Primary and Secondary Care. Clinical Guideline 23. National Institute for Health and Clinical Excellence: London.* 2007.

10. Anonymous, *Health Care Guideline: Major Depression in Adults in Primary Care. 11th edition. Institute for Clinical Systems Improvement. Available at: www.icsi.org.* 2008.

11. Dalton, S.O., et al., *Use of selective serotonin reuptake inhibitors and risk of upper gastrointestinal tract bleeding: a population-based cohort study.* Arch Intern Med, 2003. 163(1): p. 59-64.

12. Richards, J.B., et al., *Effect of selective serotonin reuptake inhibitors on the risk of fracture.* Arch Intern Med, 2007. 167(2): p. 188-94.

13. Diem, S.J., et al., *Use of antidepressants and rates of hip bone loss in older women: the study of osteoporotic fractures.* Arch Intern Med, 2007. 167(12): p. 1240-5.

14. Williams, J.W., Jr., et al., *Is this patient clinically depressed?* JAMA, 2002. 287(9): p. 1160-70.

15. Williams, J.W., Jr., *Is this patient clinically depressed?*, in *The Rational Clinical Examination: Evidence-Based Clinical Diagnosis*, S.D.L.a. Rennie, Editor. 2009, McGraw Hill. p. 247-264.

16. Gilbody, S., et al., *Screening for depression in medical settings with the Patient Health Questionnaire (PHQ): a diagnostic meta-analysis.* J Gen Intern Med, 2007. 22(11): p. 1596-602.

17. Faries, D., et al., *The responsiveness of the Hamilton Depression Rating Scale.* J Psychiatr Res, 2000. 34(1): p. 3-10.

18. Liang, M.H., A.H. Fossel, and M.G. Larson, *Comparisons of five health status instruments for orthopedic evaluation.* Med Care, 1990. 28(7): p. 632-42.

19. Deyo, R.A., P. Diehr, and D.L. Patrick, *Reproducibility and responsiveness of health status measures. Statistics and strategies for evaluation.* Control Clin Trials, 1991. 12(4 Suppl): p. 142S-158S.

20. Guyatt, G., S. Walter, and G. Norman, *Measuring change over time: assessing the usefulness of evaluative instruments.* J Chronic Dis, 1987. 40(2): p. 171-8.

21. Deyo, R.A. and R.M. Centor, *Assessing the responsiveness of functional scales to clinical change: an analogy to diagnostic test performance.* J Chronic Dis, 1986. 39(11): p. 897-906.

22. Frank, E., et al., *Conceptualization and rationale for consensus definitions of terms in major depressive disorder. Remission, recovery, relapse, and recurrence.* Arch Gen Psychiatry, 1991. 48(9): p. 851-5.

23. Panel, D.G., *Depression in Primary Care: Volume 2. Treatment of Major Depression. Clinical Practice Guideline, Number 5.*, P.H.S. U.S. Department of Health and Human Services, Agency for Health Care Policy and Research., Editor. April 1993: Rockville, MD.

24. Beck, A., R. Steer, and G. Brown, *BDI-II fast screen for medical patients manual.* 2000, London: The Psychological Corporation.

25. Andresen, E.M., et al., *Screening for depression in well older adults: evaluation of a short form of the CES-D (Center for Epidemiologic Studies Depression Scale).* Am J Prev Med, 1994. 10(2): p. 77-84.

26. Salokangas, R.K., O. Poutanen, and E. Stengard, *Screening for depression in primary care. Development and validation of the Depression Scale, a screening instrument for depression.* Acta Psychiatr Scand, 1995. 92(1): p. 10-6.

27. D'Ath, P., et al., *Screening, detection and management of depression in elderly primary care attenders. I: The acceptability and performance of the 15 item Geriatric Depression Scale (GDS15) and the development of short versions.* Fam Pract, 1994. 11(3): p. 260-6.

28. Spitzer, R.L., K. Kroenke, and J.B. Williams, *Validation and utility of a self-report version of PRIME-MD: the PHQ primary care study. Primary Care Evaluation of Mental Disorders. Patient Health Questionnaire.* JAMA, 1999. 282(18): p. 1737-44.

29. Broadhead, W.E., et al., *Development and validation of the SDDS-PC screen for multiple mental disorders in primary care.* Arch Fam Med, 1995. 4(3): p. 211-9.

30. Atkins, D., et al., *Grading quality of evidence and strength of recommendations.* Bmj, 2004. 328(7454): p. 1490.

31. Lowe, B., K. Kroenke, and K. Grafe, *Detecting and monitoring depression with a two-item questionnaire (PHQ-2).* Journal of Psychosomatic Research, 2005. 58(2): p. 163-71.

32. Lowe, B., et al., *Measuring depression outcome with a brief self-report instrument: sensitivity to change of the Patient Health Questionnaire (PHQ-9).* Journal of Affective Disorders, 2004. 81(1): p. 61-6.

33. Lowe, B., et al., *Responsiveness of the PHQ-9 to psychopharmacological depression treatment.* Psychosomatics: Journal of Consultation Liaison Psychiatry, 2006. 47(1): p. 62-67.

34. Lowe, B., et al., *Monitoring depression treatment outcomes with the patient health questionnaire-9.* Medical Care, 2004. 42(12): p. 1194-201.

35. Hansen, R., et al., *Meta-analysis of major depressive disorder relapse and recurrence with second-generation antidepressants.* Psychiatric Services, 2008. 59(10): p. 1121-30.

36. Dobson, K.S., et al., *Randomized trial of behavioral activation, cognitive therapy, and antidepressant medication in the prevention of relapse and recurrence in major depression.* Journal of Consulting and Clinical Psychology, 2008. 76(3): p. 468-77.

37. Kocsis, J.H., et al., *Prevention of recurrent episodes of depression with venlafaxine ER in a 1-year maintenance phase from the PREVENT Study.* Journal of Clinical Psychiatry, 2007.

68(7): p. 1014-23.

38. Gorwood, P., et al., *Escitalopram prevents relapse in older patients with major depressive
     disorder.* American Journal of Geriatric Psychiatry, 2007. 15(7): p. 581-93.

39. Kornstein, S.G., et al., *Assessing the efficacy of 2 years of maintenance treatment with
     venlafaxine extended release 75-225 mg/day in patients with recurrent major depression: a
     secondary analysis of data from the PREVENT study.* International Clinical Psychopharma-
     cology, 2008. 23(6): p. 357-63.

40. Kazis, L.E., J.J. Anderson, and R.F. Meenan, *Effect sizes for interpreting changes in health
     status.* Med Care, 1989. 27(3 Suppl): p. S178-89.

41. Kroenke, K., R.L. Spitzer, and J.B. Williams, *The PHQ-9: validity of a brief depression
     severity measure.* Journal of General Internal Medicine, 2001. 16(9): p. 606-13.

42. Kornstein, S.G., et al., *Escitalopram maintenance treatment for prevention of recurrent de-
     pression: a randomized, placebo-controlled trial.* J Clin Psychiatry, 2006. 67(11): p. 1767-
     75.

43. Lepine, J.P., et al., *A randomized, placebo-controlled trial of sertraline for prophylactic
     treatment of highly recurrent major depressive disorder.* Am J Psychiatry, 2004. 161(5): p.
     836-42.

44. Reimherr, F.W., et al., *Optimal length of continuation therapy in depression: a prospective
     assessment during long-term fluoxetine treatment.* Am J Psychiatry, 1998. 155(9): p. 1247-
     53.

45. Oslin, D.W., et al., *Screening, assessment, and management of depression in VA primary
     care clinics. The Behavioral Health Laboratory.* J Gen Intern Med, 2006. 21(1): p. 46-50.

46. Dowrick, C., et al., *Patients' and doctors' views on depression severity questionnaires
     incentivized in UK quality and outcomes framework: qualitative study.* BMJ, 2009. 338: p.
     b663.

47. Nease, D.E., Jr., et al., *Inducing sustainable improvement in depression care in primary care
     practices.* Jt Comm J Qual Patient Saf, 2008. 34(5): p. 247-55.

48. Duffy, F.F., et al., *Systematic use of patient-rated depression severity monitoring: is it help-
     ful and feasible in clinical psychiatry?* Psychiatr Serv, 2008. 59(10): p. 1148-54.

49. Dietrich, A.J., et al., *Re-engineering systems for the treatment of depression in primary
     care: cluster randomized controlled trial.* Bmj, 2004. 329(7466): p. 602.

50. Unutzer, J., et al., *Collaborative care management of late-life depression in the primary
     care setting: a randomized controlled trial.* JAMA, 2002. 288(22): p. 2836-45.

51. Ahava, G.W., et al., *Is the Beck Depression Inventory reliable over time? An evaluation of
     multiple test-retest reliability in a nonclinical college student sample.* Journal of Personality
     Assessment, 1998. 70(2): p. 222-31.

52. Adler, D.A., et al., *The impact of a pharmacist intervention on 6-month outcomes in de-
     pressed primary care patients.* General Hospital Psychiatry, 2004. 26(3): p. 199-209.

53. Allard, P., et al., *Efficacy and tolerability of venlafaxine in geriatric outpatients with major
     depression: a double-blind, randomized 6-month comparative trial with citalopram.* Inter-
     national Journal of Geriatric Psychiatry, 2004. 19(12): p. 1123-30.

54. Altamura, A.C., et al., *Clinical activity and tolerability of trazodone, mianserin, and ami-
     triptyline in elderly subjects with major depression: a controlled multicenter trial.* Clinical
     Neuropharmacology, 1989. 12 Suppl 1: p. S25-33; S34-7.

55. Amsterdam, J.D., J. Shults, and N. Rutherford, *Open-label study of s-citalopram therapy*

of chronic fatigue syndrome and co-morbid major depressive disorder. Progress in Neuro-Psychopharmacology and Biological Psychiatry, 2008. 32(1): p. 100-6.

56. Babyak, M., et al., *Exercise treatment for major depression: maintenance of therapeutic benefit at 10 months.* Psychosomatic Medicine, 2000. 62(5): p. 633-8.

57. Baldwin, D., R.A. Moreno, and M. Briley, *Resolution of sexual dysfunction during acute treatment of major depression with milnacipran.* Hum Psychopharmacol, 2008. 23(6): p. 527-32.

58. Barbosa, L., M. Berk, and M. Vorster, *A double-blind, randomized, placebo-controlled trial of augmentation with lamotrigine or placebo in patients concomitantly treated with fluoxetine for resistant major depressive episodes.* Journal of Clinical Psychiatry, 2003. 64(4): p. 403-7.

59. Berkman, L.F., et al., *Effects of treating depression and low perceived social support on clinical events after myocardial infarction: the Enhancing Recovery in Coronary Heart Disease Patients (ENRICHD) Randomized Trial.* JAMA, 2003. 289(23): p. 3106-16.

60. Berlim, M.T., et al., *Reliability and validity of the WHOQOL BREF in a sample of Brazilian outpatients with major depression.* Quality of Life Research, 2005. 14(2): p. 561-4.

61. Berlim, M.T., et al., *Significant improvement in the quality of life of Brazilian depressed outpatients 12 weeks following the start of antidepressants.* Psychiatry Research, 2007. 153(3): p. 253-9.

62. Boyer, P., et al., *Clinical and economic comparison of sertraline and fluoxetine in the treatment of depression. A 6-month double-blind study in a primary-care setting in France.* Pharmacoeconomics, 1998. 13(1 Pt 2): p. 157-69.

63. Brody, B.L., et al., *Age-related macular degeneration: self-management and reduction of depressive symptoms in a randomized, controlled study.* Journal of the American Geriatrics Society, 2006. 54(10): p. 1557-62.

64. Brown, C., H.C. Schulberg, and H.G. Prigerson, *Factors associated with symptomatic improvement and recovery from major depression in primary care patients.* General Hospital Psychiatry, 2000. 22(4): p. 242-50.

65. Brown, E.S., et al., *A randomized trial of citalopram versus placebo in outpatients with asthma and major depressive disorder: a proof of concept study.* Biological Psychiatry, 2005. 58(11): p. 865-70.

66. Cassidy, E.L., S. Lauderdale, and J.I. Sheikh, *Mixed anxiety and depression in older adults: clinical characteristics and management.* Journal of Geriatric Psychiatry and Neurology, 2005. 18(2): p. 83-8.

67. Casten, R.J., et al., *A comparison of self-reported function assessed before and after depression treatment among depressed geriatric patients.* International Journal of Geriatric Psychiatry, 2000. 15(9): p. 813-818.

68. Chen, T.M., et al., *Using the PHQ-9 for depression screening and treatment monitoring for Chinese Americans in primary care.* Psychiatric Services, 2006. 57(7): p. 976-81.

69. Conradi, H.J., et al., *Enhanced treatment for depression in primary care: long-term outcomes of a psycho-educational prevention program alone and enriched with psychiatric consultation or cognitive behavioral therapy.* Psychological Medicine, 2007. 37(6): p. 849-62.

70. Cook, I.A., et al., *Neurophysiologic predictors of treatment response to fluoxetine in major depression.* Psychiatry Research, 1999. 85(3): p. 263-73.

71. Corney, R. and S. Simpson, *Thirty-six month outcome data from a trial of counseling with chronically depressed patients in a general practice setting.* Psychology and Psychotherapy: Theory, Research and Practice, 2005. 78(1): p. 127-138.

72. Coulehan, J.L., et al., *Treating depressed primary care patients improves their physical, mental, and social functioning.* Archives of Internal Medicine, 1997. 157(10): p. 1113-20.

73. Dalton, E.J., et al., *Use of slow-release melatonin in treatment-resistant depression.* Journal of Psychiatry and Neuroscience, 2000. 25(1): p. 48-52.

74. Davies, J., et al., *Changes in regional cerebral blood flow with venlafaxine in the treatment of major depression.* American Journal of Psychiatry, 2003. 160(2): p. 374-6.

75. DeBattista, C., et al., *A prospective trial of bupropion SR augmentation of partial and non-responders to serotonergic antidepressants.* Journal of Clinical Psychopharmacology, 2003. 23(1): p. 27-30.

76. Dori, G.A. and J.C. Overholser, *Evaluating depression severity and remission with a modified Beck Depression Inventory.* Personality and Individual Differences, 2000. 28(6): p. 1045-1061.

77. Dubovsky, S.L., et al., *Nicardipine improves the antidepressant action of ECT but does not improve cognition.* Journal of ECT, 2001. 17(1): p. 3-10.

78. Dunner, D., et al., *Adinazolam--a new antidepressant: findings of a placebo-controlled, double-blind study in outpatients with major depression.* Journal of Clinical Psychopharmacology, 1987. 7(3): p. 170-2.

79. Einarson, T.R., *Evidence based review of escitalopram in treating major depressive disorder in primary care.* International Clinical Psychopharmacology, 2004. 19(5): p. 305-10.

80. Fava, M., et al., *Open study of the catechol-O-methyltransferase inhibitor tolcapone in major depressive disorder.* Journal of Clinical Psychopharmacology, 1999. 19(4): p. 329-35.

81. Fawcett, J., et al., *Alprazolam: an antidepressant? Alprazolam, desipramine, and an alprazolam-desipramine combination in the treatment of adult depressed outpatients.* Journal of Clinical Psychopharmacology, 1987. 7(5): p. 295-310.

82. George, T., et al., *An open study of sertraline in patients with major depression who failed to respond to moclobemide.* Australian and New Zealand Journal of Psychiatry, 1999. 33(6): p. 889-95.

83. George, T.P., et al., *Nicotinic antagonist augmentation of selective serotonin reuptake inhibitor-refractory major depressive disorder: a preliminary study.* Journal of Clinical Psychopharmacology, 2008. 28(3): p. 340-4.

84. Goodnick, P.J., et al., *Sertraline in coexisting major depression and diabetes mellitus.* Psychopharmacology Bulletin, 1997. 33(2): p. 261-4.

85. Goodnick, P.J., et al., *Bupropion slow-release response in depression: diagnosis and biochemistry.* Biological Psychiatry, 1998. 44(7): p. 629-32.

86. Judd, L.L., et al., *Randomized, placebo-controlled trial of fluoxetine for acute treatment of minor depressive disorder.* American Journal of Psychiatry, 2004. 161(10): p. 1864-71.

87. Kates, N., et al., *Counselors in primary care: benefits and lessons learned.* Canadian Journal of Psychiatry. Revue Canadienne de Psychiatrie, 2002. 47(9): p. 857-62.

88. Koivumaa-Honkanen, H., et al., *Mental health and well-being in a 6-year follow-up of patients with depression: assessments of patients and clinicians.* Social Psychiatry and Psychiatric Epidemiology, 2008. 43(9): p. 688-96.

89. Koran, L.M., et al., *Predicting response to fluoxetine in geriatric patients with major de-*

pression. Journal of Clinical Psychopharmacology, 1995. 15(6): p. 421-7.

90. Kroenke, K., et al., *Venlafaxine extended release in the short-term treatment of depressed and anxious primary care patients with multisomatoform disorder.* Journal of Clinical Psychiatry, 2006. 67(1): p. 72-80.

91. Lesperance, F., et al., *Effects of citalopram and interpersonal psychotherapy on depression in patients with coronary artery disease: the Canadian Cardiac Randomized Evaluation of Antidepressant and Psychotherapy Efficacy (CREATE) trial.* JAMA, 2007. 297(4): p. 367-79.

92. Lett, H.S., et al., *Social support and prognosis in patients at increased psychosocial risk recovering from myocardial infarction.* Health Psychology, 2007. 26(4): p. 418-427.

93. Levitt, A.J., et al., *Do depressed subjects who have failed both fluoxetine and a tricyclic antidepressant respond to the combination?* Journal of Clinical Psychiatry, 1999. 60(9): p. 613-6.

94. Liebowitz, M.R., P.P. Yeung, and R. Entsuah, *A randomized, double-blind, placebo-controlled trial of desvenlafaxine succinate in adult outpatients with major depressive disorder.* Journal of Clinical Psychiatry, 2007. 68(11): p. 1663-72.

95. Lustman, P.J., et al., *Cognitive behavior therapy for depression in type 2 diabetes mellitus. A randomized, controlled trial.* Annals of Internal Medicine, 1998. 129(8): p. 613-21.

96. Lustman, P.J., et al., *Fluoxetine for depression in diabetes: a randomized double-blind placebo-controlled trial.* Diabetes Care, 2000. 23(5): p. 618-23.

97. Lydiard, R.B., et al., *A double-blind, placebo-controlled study comparing the effects of sertraline versus amitriptyline in the treatment of major depression.* Journal of Clinical Psychiatry, 1997. 58(11): p. 484-91.

98. Mazeh, D., et al., *A randomized, single-blind, comparison of venlafaxine with paroxetine in elderly patients suffering from resistant depression.* International Clinical Psychopharmacology, 2007. 22(6): p. 371-5.

99. McIntyre, R.S., et al., *Measuring the severity of depression and remission in primary care: validation of the HAMD-7 scale.* CMAJ, 2005. 173(11): p. 1327-34.

100. Mohamed, S., et al., *Escitalopram for comorbid depression and anxiety in elderly patients: A 12-week, open-label, flexible-dose, pilot trial.* Am J Geriatr Pharmacother, 2006. 4(3): p. 201-9.

101. Mulrow, C.D., et al., *Treatment of depression--newer pharmacotherapies.* Psychopharmacology Bulletin, 1998. 34(4): p. 409-795.

102. Mynors-Wallis, L.M., et al., *Randomized controlled trial of problem solving treatment, antidepressant medication, and combined treatment for major depression in primary care.* BMJ, 2000. 320(7226): p. 26-30.

103. Patkar, A.A., et al., *A randomized, double-blind, placebo-controlled trial of augmentation with an extended release formulation of methylphenidate in outpatients with treatment-resistant depression.* Journal of Clinical Psychopharmacology, 2006. 26(6): p. 653-6.

104. Perez, V., et al., *A double-blind, randomized, placebo-controlled trial of pindolol augmentation in depressive patients resistant to serotonin reuptake inhibitors. Grup de Recerca en Trastorns Afectius.* Archives of General Psychiatry, 1999. 56(4): p. 375-9.

105. Picardi, A., et al., *Screening for depressive disorders in patients with skin diseases: a comparison of three screeners.* Acta Dermato-Venereologica, 2005. 85(5): p. 414-9.

106. Pollock, B.G., et al., *Acute antidepressant effect following pulse loading with intravenous*

and oral clomipramine. Archives of General Psychiatry, 1989. 46(1): p. 29-35.

107. Posternak, M.A. and I. Miller, *Untreated short-term course of major depression: a meta-analysis of outcomes from studies using wait-list control groups.* Journal of Affective Disorders, 2001. 66(2-3): p. 139-46.

108. Proudfoot, J., et al., *Computerized, interactive, multimedia cognitive-behavioral program for anxiety and depression in general practice.* Psychological Medicine, 2003. 33(2): p. 217-27.

109. Pyne, J.M., et al., *Use of the quality of well-being self-administered version (QWB-SA) in assessing health-related quality of life in depressed patients.* Journal of Affective Disorders, 2003. 76(1-3): p. 237-47.

110. Quilty, L.C., L.A. Meusel, and R.M. Bagby, *Neuroticism as a mediator of treatment response to SSRIs in major depressive disorder.* Journal of Affective Disorders, 2008. 111(1): p. 67-73.

111. Raskin, J., et al., *Duloxetine in the long-term treatment of major depressive disorder.* Journal of Clinical Psychiatry, 2003. 64(10): p. 1237-44.

112. Raskin, J., et al., *Efficacy of duloxetine on cognition, depression, and pain in elderly patients with major depressive disorder: an 8-week, double-blind, placebo-controlled trial.* American Journal of Psychiatry, 2007. 164(6): p. 900-9.

113. Rollman, B.L., et al., *A randomized trial using computerized decision support to improve treatment of major depression in primary care.* Journal of General Internal Medicine, 2002. 17(7): p. 493-503.

114. Rush, A.J. and A. Bose, *Escitalopram in clinical practice: results of an open-label trial in a naturalistic setting.* Depression and Anxiety, 2005. 21(1): p. 26-32.

115. Rutherford, B., et al., *An open trial of aripiprazole augmentation for SSRI non-remitters with late-life depression.* International Journal of Geriatric Psychiatry, 2007. 22(10): p. 986-91.

116. Salkovskis, P., et al., *A randomized controlled trial of the use of self-help materials in addition to standard general practice treatment of depression compared to standard treatment alone.* Psychological Medicine, 2006. 36(3): p. 325-33.

117. Shelton, R.C., et al., *Effectiveness of St John's wort in major depression: a randomized controlled trial.* JAMA, 2001. 285(15): p. 1978-86.

118. Singh, N.A., K.M. Clements, and M.A. Singh, *The efficacy of exercise as a long-term antidepressant in elderly subjects: a randomized, controlled trial.* Journals of Gerontology. Series A, Biological Sciences and Medical Sciences, 2001. 56(8): p. M497-504.

119. Skevington, S.M. and A. Wright, *Changes in the quality of life of patients receiving antidepressant medication in primary care: Validation of the WHOQOL-100.* British Journal of Psychiatry, 2001. 178: p. 261-267.

120. Spalletta, G., A. Pasini, and C. Caltagirone, *Fluoxetine alone in the treatment of first episode anxious-depression: an open clinical trial.* Journal of Clinical Psychopharmacology, 2002. 22(3): p. 263-6.

121. Stark, P. and C.D. Hardison, *A review of multicenter controlled studies of fluoxetine vs. imipramine and placebo in outpatients with major depressive disorder.* Journal of Clinical Psychiatry, 1985. 46(3 Pt 2): p. 53-8.

122. Szegedi, A., et al., *Acute treatment of moderate to severe depression with hypericum extract WS 5570 (St John's wort): randomized controlled double blind non-inferiority trial versus*

paroxetine. BMJ, 2005. 330(7490): p. 503.

123. Thase, M.E., *Efficacy and tolerability of once-daily venlafaxine extended release (XR) in outpatients with major depression. The Venlafaxine XR 209 Study Group.* Journal of Clinical Psychiatry, 1997. 58(9): p. 393-8.

124. Trivedi, M.H., et al., *Clinical results for patients with major depressive disorder in the Texas Medication Algorithm Project.* Archives of General Psychiatry, 2004. 61(7): p. 669-80.

125. Tutty, S., G. Simon, and E. Ludman, *Telephone counseling as an adjunct to antidepressant treatment in the primary care system. A pilot study.* Effective Clinical Practice, 2000. 3(4): p. 170-8.

126. van Gurp, G., et al., *St John's wort or sertraline? Randomized controlled trial in primary care.* Canadian Family Physician, 2002. 48: p. 905-12.

127. van Marwijk, H.W., et al., *Primary care management of major depression in patients aged > or =55 years: outcome of a randomized clinical trial.* British Journal of General Practice, 2008. 58(555): p. 680-6, I-II; discussion 687.

128. Vinkers, D.J., et al., *The 15-item Geriatric Depression Scale (GDS-15) detects changes in depressive symptoms after a major negative life event. The Leiden 85-plus Study.* International Journal of Geriatric Psychiatry, 2004. 19(1): p. 80-4.

129. Wade, A.G., et al., *Escitalopram and duloxetine in major depressive disorder: a pharmaco-economic comparison using UK cost data.* Pharmacoeconomics, 2008. 26(11): p. 969-81.

130. Wise, T.N., et al., *The safety and tolerability of duloxetine in depressed elderly patients with and without medical comorbidity.* International Journal of Clinical Practice, 2007. 61(8): p. 1283-93.

131. Bauer, M., et al., *The effect of venlafaxine compared with other antidepressants and placebo in the treatment of major depression: A meta-analysis.* European Archives of Psychiatry and Clinical Neuroscience, 2009.

132. Gartlehner, G., et al., *Comparative benefits and harms of second-generation antidepressants: background paper for the American College of Physicians.* Annals of Internal Medicine, 2008. 149(10): p. 734-50.

133. Qaseem, A., et al., *Using second-generation antidepressants to treat depressive disorders: a clinical practice guideline from the American College of Physicians.* Annals of Internal Medicine, 2008. 149(10): p. 725-33.

134. Anderson, I.M., et al., *Evidence-based guidelines for treating depressive disorders with antidepressants: a revision of the 2000 British Association for Psychopharmacology guidelines.* J Psychopharmacol, 2008. 22(4): p. 343-96.

135. Papakostas, G.I., et al., *Antidepressant dose reduction and the risk of relapse in major depressive disorder.* Psychotherapy and Psychosomatics, 2007. 76(5): p. 266-70.

136. Furukawa, T.A., et al., *Long-term treatment of depression with antidepressants: a systematic narrative review.* Canadian Journal of Psychiatry. Revue Canadienne de Psychiatrie, 2007. 52(9): p. 545-52.

137. Zimmerman, M., M.A. Posternak, and C.J. Ruggero, *Impact of study design on the results of continuation studies of antidepressants.* Journal of Clinical Psychopharmacology, 2007. 27(2): p. 177-81.

138. Lam, R.W. and S.H. Kennedy, *Evidence-based strategies for achieving and sustaining full remission in depression: focus on metaanalyses.* Canadian Journal of Psychiatry. Revue

Canadienne de Psychiatrie, 2004. 49(3 Suppl 1): p. 17S-26S.

139. Dombrovski, A.Y., et al., *Maintenance treatment for old-age depression preserves health-related quality of life: a randomized, controlled trial of paroxetine and interpersonal psychotherapy.* Journal of the American Geriatrics Society, 2007. 55(9): p. 1325-32.

140. Keller, M.B., et al., *The Prevention of Recurrent Episodes of Depression with Venlafaxine for Two Years (PREVENT) Study: Outcomes from the 2-year and combined maintenance phases.* Journal of Clinical Psychiatry, 2007. 68(8): p. 1246-56.

141. Doogan, D.P. and V. Caillard, *Sertraline in the prevention of depression.* Br J Psychiatry, 1992. 160: p. 217-22.

142. Feiger, A.D., et al., *Double-blind, placebo-substitution study of nefazodone in the prevention of relapse during continuation treatment of outpatients with major depression.* Int Clin Psychopharmacol, 1999. 14(1): p. 19-28.

143. Gelenberg, A.J., et al., *Randomized, placebo-controlled trial of nefazodone maintenance treatment in preventing recurrence in chronic depression.* Biol Psychiatry, 2003. 54(8): p. 806-17.

144. Gilaberte, I., et al., *Fluoxetine in the prevention of depressive recurrences: a double-blind study.* J Clin Psychopharmacol, 2001. 21(4): p. 417-24.

145. Hochstrasser, B., et al., *Prophylactic effect of citalopram in unipolar, recurrent depression: placebo-controlled study of maintenance therapy.* Br J Psychiatry, 2001. 178: p. 304-10.

146. Keller, M.B., et al., *Maintenance phase efficacy of sertraline for chronic depression: a randomized controlled trial.* JAMA, 1998. 280(19): p. 1665-72.

147. Klysner, R., et al., *Efficacy of citalopram in the prevention of recurrent depression in elderly patients: placebo-controlled study of maintenance therapy.* Br J Psychiatry, 2002. 181: p. 29-35.

148. Lustman, P.J., et al., *Sertraline for prevention of depression recurrence in diabetes mellitus: a randomized, double-blind, placebo-controlled trial.* Arch Gen Psychiatry, 2006. 63(5): p. 521-9.

149. Montgomery, S.A., J.G. Rasmussen, and P. Tanghoj, *A 24-week study of 20 mg citalopram, 40 mg citalopram, and placebo in the prevention of relapse of major depression.* Int Clin Psychopharmacol, 1993. 8(3): p. 181-8.

150. Montgomery, S.A., et al., *Venlafaxine versus placebo in the preventive treatment of recurrent major depression.* J Clin Psychiatry, 2004. 65(3): p. 328-36.

151. Montgomery, S.A. and G. Dunbar, *Paroxetine is better than placebo in relapse prevention and the prophylaxis of recurrent depression.* Int Clin Psychopharmacol, 1993. 8(3): p. 189-95.

152. Reynolds, C.F., 3rd, et al., *Maintenance treatment of major depression in old age.* N Engl J Med, 2006. 354(11): p. 1130-8.

153. Robert, P. and S.A. Montgomery, *Citalopram in doses of 20-60 mg is effective in depression relapse prevention: a placebo-controlled 6 month study.* Int Clin Psychopharmacol, 1995. 10 Suppl 1: p. 29-35.

154. Schmidt, M.E., et al., *The efficacy and safety of a new enteric-coated formulation of fluoxetine given once weekly during the continuation treatment of major depressive disorder.* J Clin Psychiatry, 2000. 61(11): p. 851-7.

155. Simon, J.S., et al., *Extended-release venlafaxine in relapse prevention for patients with major depressive disorder.* J Psychiatr Res, 2004. 38(3): p. 249-57.

156. Terra, J.L. and S.A. Montgomery, *Fluvoxamine prevents recurrence of depression: results of a long-term, double-blind, placebo-controlled study.* Int Clin Psychopharmacol, 1998. 13(2): p. 55-62.

157. Thase, M.E., et al., *Efficacy of mirtazapine for prevention of depressive relapse: a placebo-controlled double-blind trial of recently remitted high-risk patients.* J Clin Psychiatry, 2001. 62(10): p. 782-8.

158. Weihs, K.L., et al., *Continuation phase treatment with bupropion SR effectively decreases the risk for relapse of depression.* Biol Psychiatry, 2002. 51(9): p. 753-61.

159. Wilson, K.C., et al., *Older community residents with depression: long-term treatment with sertraline. Randomized, double-blind, placebo-controlled study.* Br J Psychiatry, 2003. 182: p. 492-7.

www.ingramcontent.com/pod-product-compliance
Lightning Source LLC
Chambersburg PA
CBHW081615170526
45166CB00009B/2980